TH. SLIM DAYS

Create your slender and healthy life in a fun and enjoyable way

FIONA FERRIS

ISBN- 13: 978-1544171944
ISBN- 10: 1544171943

Book Bonuses

bit.ly/FreeBookBonuses

Go to the link above to receive your free special bonuses – book excerpts and other chic goodies.

You will also **receive a subscription** to Fiona's blog *'How to be Chic'*, for weekly inspiration on living a simple and beautiful life.

Contents

Introduction

I think it's fair to say that most of us already know the nuts and bolts to losing weight and maintaining slimness... in theory. It is likely we all know to:

Eat healthily
Keep processed foods to a minimum
Have treat foods sparingly
Drink plenty of fluids such as water and herbal tea
Don't take in too much caffeine
Sleep well by having consistent wake and sleep times
Lower stress levels as much as possible

So what's stopping us doing *that*, instead of spending all our time and energy following diets, reading this book (writing this book!), going for the next quick fix, despairing over our clothes not fitting yet eating more to feel better?

It's something I have pondered a lot over the years; I mean, how hard can it be to eat normally and be a normal weight? To peacefully co-exist with food? What was wrong with me that I could not get this one part of my life right?

The answer my friends, is M I N D S E T.

Since the day we were born we have absorbed the views of those closest to us about what we eat and why we eat.

If you haven't intentionally changed what you think, you are probably eating the same kinds of meals and treat foods now that you did when you were living with your parents and siblings.

Even television programs we watched growing up have shaped our beliefs. Where else did we learn that if a boy dumps us or a friend betrays us, that we will feel better eating a container of ice-cream sitting on our bed crying?

Each of us has our own tangled and complicated version of what type and quantity of food we believe is acceptable to eat; our own beliefs of what our weight could be and how we feel about food and eating in general.

If I asked myself in the past what I believed about food, I would have said:

I often don't have control over what I eat
I let my cravings lead me
I wish I could eat normally but I can't seem to
My sweet tooth rules everything
Now that I am over forty, I can't lose weight

Examining these statements individually, I found that they were not facts; but simply thoughts I had been thinking for so long that I now believed they were true for me. Instead of continuing to live by them, I decided to view this as a golden opportunity to change my beliefs now I knew what they were.

I have heard the saying 'diets don't work' many times. That always confused me, because it was obvious that if I ate less and better, I would become slimmer. The missing part for me was that this would be okay if we were robots; but we are human beings with emotions, memories and feelings.

Diets address the outside world – what we are eating – but they do nothing to change the inside world – our mindset. Changing the outside world brings the novelty of something new, plus willpower works for a while; but then our mind will snap us back to what we were doing before, because the changes we made were superficial.

Our minds are lazy, they like comfort and staying the same. To keep this status quo, our minds can actively sabotage us if we try to change too quickly, even if the changes are better for us and we are happy with them.

I found that a new diet worked well to start with; I was full of enthusiasm for a change and thrilled when the weight started coming off. But after a while – it could even be quite a long time – something happened. I would stand by helplessly as the weight came back on. It was horrible to experience but I felt powerless to stop it.

What helped me stay with my new healthy eating regime was working on my slim mindset at the same time. With my journey to feeling peaceful around eating, I found that I needed constant inspiration and encouragement, especially in the beginning.

Sometimes one trick that had worked for a while stopped working so well for me and I found myself slipping back into old habits. So I started devising a chic toolkit of sorts that I could dip into whenever I needed the motivation.

I have so many techniques in my toolkit now, that if I fall off the wagon I can pick myself up so much quicker than I used to. As a result, my eating (and my weight) is much more stable and therefore healthier. I also have a wonderful peace of mind around food, that I did not have before.

I used to think there was one thing. One thing that would flick the switch for me. I was chasing around solutions that I expected to fix everything once and for all. Time after time I was disappointed and I began to doubt myself.

Maybe I wasn't fixable? Was I was destined to be a slave to my sweet tooth and never be able to wear my lovely smaller-sized clothes again? Was I going to descend into middle age a dumpy frump?

That sort of downward spiral did not feel good. And it was caused by unhelpful thoughts from a little doubting voice inside of me that *were not even true*. They were fears and worries, not fact.

I work on loving myself exactly as I am regardless of what I weigh or how I look. But does this have to exclude me being my best self? Why not claim both? There's no law that says you must do one or the other.

And what's the alternative? Continuing to get a little bit heavier each year until I develop health issues? Feeling bad about myself because I know I could look and feel so much better than I do?

If you loved yourself, you would naturally want to nourish your body with good food, wouldn't you? If you loved a family member, you would want to serve them good meals and treat them in a loving way. Would you force them to eat junk food until they felt ill? Of course not! But for me, that's exactly what I was doing.

Something was out of sync, and once I started working on my mindset with all the techniques in the following chapters, I realized I could find my way back to my happy weight – gently, patiently and lovingly.

Of course, I knew I needed to change the way I ate, but having the right mindset helped me keep on going and not give up at the first hurdle (or craving). The great news is that eating well and looking after yourself becomes easier over time. It becomes your new normal. I know from personal experience that if you can get your food thoughts under control, it releases so much mental energy and you are set free to start living your life; instead of spending much of the day thinking about food and eating; trying to eat normally and feeling out of control.

Even if you have been losing weight and loving the way you look and feel, you may find yourself slipping back into old habits and eating the foods you have been avoiding to lose weight. I've done it myself many times and it is so frustrating. You feel weak-willed, a failure and like you will *never* be your ideal weight. You consider that it must be your destiny to always be struggling with weight loss and eating too much.

There is a saying I love: *If the front door is locked, go in through the window; if the window is shut, try the side gate.* That's how I find success with anything I wish to do, and especially being at my ideal weight and feeling happy and healthy. I approach it from all directions and I never give up.

Everything included in this book is designed to change your mindset in lots of little ways, from many different angles. If you make small enough changes and have them bed in as 'just what you do', the 'I don't want to change, I'm comfortable the way I am' part of your brain will not be triggered.

It doesn't matter if you will always be a work in progress regarding healthy eating and subsequent slimness. If you are making more steps forward than back, you can consider yourself a success. You will always win as long as keep going.

I also do not believe you have to be *at* your goal weight to consider yourself a success. If you are making progress, and feel happy and calm within yourself as you go about your day, eating in a natural and healthy way; you are a success right now.

Have you heard that cheesy motivational saying 'Quitters never win, and winners never quit'? I love that saying, and it helps me get through a tough day of cravings or when I can't be bothered planning healthy meals. It helps me keep on going.

As with my first book *Thirty Chic Days*, this book is set up into thirty distinct chapters, or 'days'. You can read *Thirty Slim Days* chronologically, or you may choose to read different chapters as they appeal to you.

This book isn't a typical diet book with a list of rules, to-dos and meal plans. I hope that it won't be dry or bossy or prescriptive. My goal for this book is to be happy, inspiring, encouraging and a little bit silly at times; because when we get too serious, we stop listening.

If we can put a little bit of frivolity and inspiration into the process of becoming our ideal weight, we are more likely to follow up and get there. Why would we want to do something if it isn't fun?

And the bonus of making the process enjoyable is that we won't even have noticed that we are eating different foods, partaking in different activities and losing weight in a more effortless way.

Most people don't get to and stay at their goal weight because they make it into a big ordeal, then give up too soon; it's as simple as that. I know you are not one of those people – you are focused on doing whatever it takes to upgrade this area of your life. It doesn't have to be hard, but you do have to be focused. You keep on going, no matter what.

I am so excited for you, just as I am excited for myself continuing this journey. Today is a new day, a fresh new start; perfect for you to start living a life of freedom, happiness and good health.

Here's to you.

Day 1
My story

I wasn't overweight as a child, but I certainly loved my food. We had normal, healthy home-cooked meals, and treats at the weekend. Once I started earning my own money at high school, this progressed to treats most days because I loved them so much. Doing this caught up with me in my late teens and this is when I joined a gym for the first time.

In my mid-twenties, I tried Weight Watchers and fell into the low-fat, high-carb way of thinking. I read Susan Powter's book *Stop The Insanity!* over and over. 'Fat makes you fat' was the message, so you could eat endless amounts of low-fat foods and still be skinny, or so Susan said.

Today I know better, I know it is not true; yet it was so ingrained in me at the time, I still have this thought that I can eat anything I like, in any quantity as long as it is low-fat. *To this day* I still believe deep down that a bag of candy is harmless because it is non-fat. And I know all about insulin! Some information – even if it is erroneous – really sticks around.

It's as if I constantly have to re-remember. I have never had a proper eating disorder (that I know of), but I truly believe that my disordered thinking around food and eating comes from those diet days. My love of sweet foods goes way back though, to when I was less than ten years old. I enjoyed candy, ice-cream and party food, probably like a lot of children do.

You're given them as treats because your parents want you to have a bit of fun, but some of us take it right through to adulthood with us and don't know how to deal with it. We recreate good times and happiness by eating the foods that made us feel happy and loved when we were younger.

In my twenties, I became a bit frumpy looking and that's when I started my first proper diet, Weight Watchers, as I mentioned before. My kids party food habit had caught up with me. I signed up and the weight started dropping off. I thought, *This is it, this is the answer*, but once the novelty and enthusiasm of beginning a diet wore off, the subconscious beliefs and my old way of being came back to the surface. I was hungry and worn down and the weight piled back on.

I also received mixed messages about my weight and food choices. I said to someone close to me once that I'd lost some weight and they said 'oh that's great, you don't look so fat anymore' and other comments like that, so it let me know that I needed to lose a bit of weight.

Then, when I was careful, trying to eat low-fat or low-carb, depending on the trend of the time; I was made to feel like I was being faddy, making a fuss and calling attention to myself. It was very subtle, but it made me feel like crap.

It also makes you second-guess yourself and doubt what you're doing. I know I'm not alone in this; I think it's such a common scenario for women. I had such a messed-up view of my body and how it 'should' be perfect.

Thinking back, for all my adult life I have been conscious of my weight – either trying to get it down, or revelling in a temporary weight loss and subsequently wearing my favourite small-size clothes. If I count the years, it's been more than twenty-five years that I have had that drain on my thinking.

Can you relate? Do you have a similar story?

Imagine if you simply went about your day in a normal and carefree manner, eating what you knew was tasty and healthy and not giving it a second thought until it came time to prepare your next meal. Imagine how much mental space and energy would be freed up to do other things.

In some ways you may feel sad about the time and energy wasted, but you can't change the past. Instead, put a positive spin on it. You can choose to feel excited for a future where you are unshackled from this way of thinking. You know that you have made life harder for yourself than it needed to be. Now, you see it is now fully within your control to effect the change you desire.

In the past you have acted how you have because of the information and knowledge you had at the time. Your mind is like a computer where the programming dictates how you act. Imagine if you could change the programming; you wouldn't have to try to eat healthier, avoid unhealthy foods and exercise more. It would become effortless and something you wouldn't even have to think about.

That's what I had been searching for all along. If you asked me, I'd know in theory what a slim and healthy person ate and how they behaved. But I didn't want that solution; I wanted my favourite snack foods to be calorie-free and healthy.

I used to wish that sweet and salty popcorn could be a complete food group so that it was an acceptable meal choice. I would dream that all the foods I loved to stuff myself with would magically become good for me and salads would be bad.

But I was arguing with reality, which meant I was going to lose one-hundred-percent of the time. There was nothing I could do to make unhealthy foods healthier.

I was half-way right though – the trick to enjoying your favourite foods while still being slim and healthy is to *change what your favourite foods are*. Reprogram your mind about what foods are a treat for you. Then eating in a healthful manner becomes easy.

When you change the programming underneath, it means nutritious eating and moving in a way that supports your health becomes your new normal, no willpower necessary. Wouldn't that be incredible? Actually wanting to eat a bright salad and lean protein for lunch instead of something stodgy? Being happy with one drink before dinner and no salty nibbles?

For me, it wasn't just about following a diet, but working out what was going on in my mind as well. I often wished I had a toolkit of all the techniques that had worked for me in the past so that I could dip in and out of them as required. I have been recording them and re-testing them and this book is a result of that.

Let's begin.

Day 2
Start with a vision

Would you like to know the best way to bring your dream slim life to you, today? It's simple and so easy that you may already know how, or if you didn't before will wonder how it wasn't obvious to you already.

The goal of becoming your happy weight – and easily staying there in a healthy manner – is easy to accept. Who wouldn't choose that? But wanting that outcome and having it come true are two different things. To achieve your goal, you need to prepare your mind by developing a detailed picture of the future; otherwise how will you know when you have arrived?

Lots of people have a goal weight, but they have no idea of how their life will look when they are that person living at a lower weight. They won't be doing the same things they are now but that's all they know; and they might not even know that. They might expect that they can continue exactly as they are now, and that the fat fairy will grant them their wish overnight.

Something to consider when dreaming of your slim future is:

How will your daily routines look compared to now?
Your meals?
The way you move?
Does your home look different?
Who do you live with?

The best way to have exactly what you want to happen, is to craft a vision of your dream slim and healthy life; paint a picture of how your days will be when your goals have happened.

Doing this is the first step in becoming the new you; the 2.0 version who easily reaches her goal weight in a fun and easy way, then effortlessly maintains that weight consistently.

You will start attracting your ideal slim future to you both in the way you think of it, and also by implementing tiny changes that you can see the new you doing. *Become a visionary of your life.* See things not as they are but as they could be.

I know it sounds simplistic and like wishful thinking, but it really works. Regularly, I will take the time to daydream and brainwash myself into all the ways in which my life will be even more wonderful than it already is. I think about how slim and healthy I am and how I go through a typical day. Before too long, I am living more and more of that dream life as my actual, real, right-now life.

How would you spend your perfect day?

One of my favourite ways to do this is to come up with my perfect day. A day in which I had everything I always wanted and spent it doing whatever I wanted.

Spend some time with your journal and write out your ideal day – doing two is helpful; one is your ideal work day and the other is your ideal home day, play day or vacation day. Write out your ideal days like you are watching a movie with yourself as the main character. Doing this helps you bring up your ideal work and play scenarios.

I would heartily recommend this little project; it doesn't have to take long and if you don't fancy yourself much of a writer, you can note down bullet points. These are some of my examples that I have written. I love this exercise so much!

One of my normal days...

I wake up at 6am with the alarm and spring out of bed. I weigh myself and see that my weight is the same low number. I used to think it would be a dream to wake up skinny and now I do, because I went to bed skinny. I had a fantastic night's sleep as I always do these days. No more tossing and turning from all that sugar in my system.

After feeding the cats and making myself a cup of tea, I get straight into my writing. I love writing first thing in the morning and find that I do my best work, so I always make sure not to open anything else on my browser at this time.

After two hours of writing and maybe another cup of tea, I put my leggings and tee-shirt on and go for a brisk walk around the neighbourhood. It's a lovely time of the day and I see dogs being walked and children being taken to school. Once or twice a week I will do a yoga class instead of going for a walk.

I arrive back home and take a shower before my breakfast of fresh fruits, overnight oats and yoghurt with cinnamon, and a soy café latte to finish. I'll do another hour or two or writing and then it is time for lunch. I have a big salad with avocado and leftover roast chicken with a sprinkle of lemon juice or dressing, then a piece of fruit for afters.

In the afternoon I do some errands, maybe buy groceries and do my housework. Mid- to late-afternoon I have recognised as the point in my day when I have the least energy or motivation, so I look forward to reading a book for an hour or so and sometimes even have a small nap.

Later on I cook a quick and healthy meal of fresh oven-baked fish and steamed vegetables which are dressed in lemon-infused olive oil. A squeeze of lemon juice, and dinner is served. I finish off with a bliss ball and a small decaf coffee and watch an episode of my current television program before heading off to our bedroom for my boudoir time.

I switch on soft spa music and potter around washing my face, applying a mask and smoothing my heels before moisturizing with body cream. I flick through a Victoria magazine while I wait for my mask to dry, then rinse it off; my warm damp skin ready for serum and night cream.

Settling into bed with a book to read I reflect on my simple, healthy and fulfilling day; giving grace for my beautiful life. Thank you.

This day is pretty much my normal day now, but it wasn't when I imagined it at first. By dreaming of it and re-reading it often, I gradually took the steps towards that ideal day and now I am there, which I am very happy and grateful for.

For the longest time when I couldn't fit the smallest clothes in my closet, I had this beautiful daydream that one day when... One day when I was slim and felt confident and could wear anything at all from my closet with ease, I imagined myself on a trip to Paris.

This vision kept me going, kept me trying method after method to click my mindset so that it could come true.

Here is my vision:

A day in Paris...

My darling and I arrived in Paris two days ago, and today we are doing what we always talked about – strolling the streets of Paris as if we were locals. We are going to find a café not far from our building for breakfast, and then spend the rest of the day exploring.

I open my armoire where I have hung my travel wardrobe and choose my clothes for the day. It's a little chillier so I am wearing my mid-wash skinny jeans. They are Diesel jeans and I have had them for quite a while, but they are almost new. Why is that, you ask?

Well, I bought them and then grew out of them. I had to put them aside for a couple of years but now I fit them with ease. They slide up my legs and fit snugly around my hips and waist. I don't have to wear a belt with them because they have a mid-cut waist so they won't slide down.

I've always wanted to be able to wear a tight pair of jeans with a tee-shirt sitting flatly across the waistband – no overhang or muffin-top! – and now I do, all the time. This fabulous feeling never grows old.

With my skinny jeans I wear a black and white striped boat-neck top with bracelet-length sleeves (my favourite neckline and sleeve length). I know it sounds clichéd to wear a Breton-style top in Paris, but I don't care.

Over that I wear a black blazer with a nipped-in waist and chunky black New Balance trainers. I love that the athleisure trend makes it easier to dress stylishly when you are a tourist!

I blow-dried my hair straight yesterday so I brush it carefully and apply light makeup from my minimal travel collection – long-wear foundation applied sheerly with a damp sponge, a dusting of powder to set it, pretty pink blush, lip balm and lashings of mascara with my favourite Mac eyeshadow in Velux Kid. To finish, I shape my eyebrows with dark brown powder and a brush.

I grab my small cross-body bag and off we go to experience our Parisian life. We walk down the steps from our rental apartment onto the street and it is just like we dreamed of. The scooters, the stylish Parisians starting their day, the baguettes. Such a thrill!

Settling in at a café, I feel like I belong. I am not self-conscious about my stomach rolling over my waistband when I sit down and I feel comfortable and happy. I know I will find gorgeous little boutiques during our wanderings today and when I try clothes on, they will look great on me. I won't come out of changing rooms dejected like I used to, because I am happy with what I see in the mirror whether I am clothed or in my underwear.

Thank you. Life is good!

I don't know about you, but I found myself drifting into the reverie of those two days. It felt like I was right there; and that's a good thing, because it means I am playing a movie to my mind, and my mind doesn't know that those movies are not true for me... yet.

Your perfect days are highly likely to be different to mine. Your vacation day might be you enjoying your resort holiday in Mexico, relaxing on the sun lounger in your retro bikini while your children play in the pool just beyond your toes. You look down at your slim physique as you sip a cool coconut drink and see that your husband is making eyes at you from behind his aviators...

Build little details like that into your dream days and they will touch your emotions, which is how you can change your mindset easily. Our mind loves emotion. If you look at a picture, you will see it and appreciate it. But if you look at a picture while conjuring up an emotion, your mind will accept it much more readily.

Notice how both of my dream days don't have me spending two hours at the gym or eating tiny portions of rabbit food. I don't wish to live that way, so I don't. The secret to becoming slender in a happy way is to build your slim life as you wish to experience it.

Diets never worked long term for me because I would knuckle down and be strict for a short time then go back to the way I was before. The strictness was not sustainable. Result: yoyo dieting and an unhappy Fiona.

Take your time and enjoy the journey

Now, I happily go slower as I build new habits and supportive structure into my days. I am living the way I can see myself being for the rest of my life. I lost my weight the slowest I ever have – a mere one kilogram or two pounds a month, but it was for good this time so I didn't care if it didn't happen quickly. It's slower to decrease my weight but it is sustainable because I am building new habits based on my vision.

In the end it comes down to the small things, and asking yourself, *If I wanted to create this sort of life for myself, this happiness with my slim physique, what are the small achievable habits I need?*

Then start slotting them into your everyday life. Because the future you? She is created today and every day. She **is** today. Today is your future because there is no tomorrow. Tomorrow will be today once it gets here. It sounds like an *Alice in Wonderland* riddle, but it's the truth.

When I got that, everything changed for me. I could no longer kid myself about all the rubbish I used to eat, thinking, *But I want it now, I'll be good tomorrow.* Once tomorrow arrived, I'd put it off again.

When I got that today is the only day I had, I started to make better choices and made it fun to make better choices. Create your perfect day to bring your future to you right now, to see what bright and shining experience you have to look forward to. Happiness is right around the corner.

Your *Thirty Slim Days* action tips:

Write or type out your perfect days. **Include lots of glorious detail** about how and what you eat; how you feel about food (good, peaceful, in control) and how amazing it is to choose your clothes that fit you well each morning. Soak it all in.

Read your perfect days often and **conjure up all those good feelings** as you picture how wonderful life is at your happy weight. Feel as if it has already happened and you will be well on your way.

Day 3

Start your 'slender you' notebook

When I became serious about resetting my eating habits, I began with a new notebook. This notebook was small enough that I could use one page per day and I wrote on both sides of the paper. It is an A5 size which is the equivalent of size US 5.83" X 8.27" paper, just to give you an idea.

On page one I wrote the date, 'Day 1' and my weight. I noted everything down that I ate for the day; and I often I wrote down what I was going to eat before the meal, because I had already planned my menu.

If I was particularly organized, and especially in the beginning, I wrote out my day's meal plan the night before. This made sure I had all the necessary fresh ingredients and the next day I didn't have to make any decisions; I just had to follow what was listed.

I often found it easier to detach myself from the next day's menu and plan it out as if I was the personal household chef and it was my job to ensure that my client had a day of healthy and nutritious food that would give her the energy to get through her day.

Because I had always snacked, my meals sometimes weren't that big which meant I was legitimately snacking because I was getting hungry; the issue was that my snacks were not often good choices.

I wasn't trying to eat small meals, but I was trying to eat healthily. I was serious about trying to eat three meals a day with *no snacks*, so my meals had to be big enough to get me through to the next meal.

I wanted to get out of the habit of snacking for good, because I knew three strict meals a day was a much better habit for me personally. There is more about this in the chapter '*Day 12. Become someone who does not snack*'.

I weighed myself daily. Looking at my weight on the scales does not worry me; it's simply an interesting fact for the day. If weighing yourself messes with your head, weigh less often; maybe monthly to keep an eye on progress without focusing on it too much. Make sure you note it on day one though, as a starting point.

Let yourself be supported and encouraged

I kept this whole process as transparent as possible, and had my notebook lying open (it was spiral-bound) on the kitchen counter most the time. I didn't mind that my husband could see it whenever I wrote my weight at the top of that day's page, and he was very supportive.

Talk about your goal with your spouse; get them on board. I mentioned to my husband that I was being a little stricter with myself, but that we would still be having our usual meals. I was planning to tweak mine a bit – having as many green vegetables as before, but measuring my protein, fat and starchy vegetables to make sure I was getting the right amounts.

My pattern used to be that I was not getting enough protein but too many starchy carbs. Measuring helped keep this in check. In my notebook I wrote if I had measured something, otherwise I just noted 'steamed and roasted vegetables' on a line.

Here is a sample day from my food notebook:

First thing in the morning:
Hot tea with trim milk, no sugar

Breakfast:
6 oz. fresh chopped fruit
1 piece of gluten-free toast with peanut butter and
*   apricot jam on top*
4 oz. soy milk café latte

Lunch:
6 oz. raw, fresh mixed salad vegetables (lettuce,
*   tomato, zucchini/courgette, red onion)*

3 oz. cold meat chopped up (dinner leftovers)
½ oz. raw almonds/pumpkin seeds
2 oz. avocado
Lemon juice squirted over to dress
A bliss ball
Coffee with trim milk (unsweetened)

Pre-dinner:
Lemon Perrier sparkling water

Dinner – we had homemade roast dinner, so:
4 oz. roast chicken
Roasted vegetables – a slice of pumpkin, half an onion, half a carrot
Steamed broccoli and green beans with a dash of olive oil to dress
Pan dripping gravy made with gravy mix and a sprinkle of dried sage
A square of Lindt 90% cacao chocolate
Earl Grey tea with trim milk, unsweetened

Choose a way to lose weight that you can live with forever

As time passed, my initial regime had become less strict and I started adding in little extras. The sample day above includes items I did not have in the beginning, namely toast, peanut butter and jam, bliss ball and dark chocolate.

I didn't see this as cheating, because my whole goal in becoming slim was doing it in a way that I could happily carry on with for the rest of my life. Unlike other efforts in the past, I did not want a crash diet or a quick fix.

By starting off strictly and then blending it into how I could see myself continuing, I gave myself the best chance of success. I had reset my eating habits, because they were a little out of kilter veering on the side of wanton excess; and I then loosened my parameters a bit so that I didn't feel trapped in diet jail.

Borrow inspiration to encourage you

I love reading slimming quotes daily as motivation. Some of my favourite quotes that I have noted down over the years are:

'If you want to change you have to be willing to be uncomfortable'.
(by this I take that the uncomfortableness of not being able to eat chocolate every afternoon, not that I am going to starve myself)

'Out of sight, out of mind. Out of the house, out of my stomach.'

'If you want to see changes, you have to make changes.'

'If no one else does, I still will.'

'Discipline is remembering what you want.'

'Motivation is like food for the brain. You cannot get enough in one sitting. It needs continual and regular top ups.'

'Bigger snacks mean bigger slacks.'

'If hunger is not the problem, then eating is not the solution.'

'Another good reducing exercise consists in placing both hands against the table edge and pushing back.'

'Your body keeps an accurate journal regardless of what you write down.'

'A year from now, you may wish you had started today.'

'The greatest thing you have is the twenty-four hours in front of you. The past is gone; the future is distant. Today you can succeed. Set a goal you can achieve in the next twenty-four hours.'

'The best thing about the future is that it only comes one day at a time.'

'It's the little details that are vital. Little things make big things happen.'

'Rather than aiming for perfect, aim to be a little bit better today than you were yesterday.'

'Your past does not equal, nor does it dictate, your future.'

'What you eat in private, you wear in public.'

'Don't dream it, be it.'

'You haven't failed until you have given up trying.'

'Nothing changes if nothing changes.'

As I progressed through my notebook and started loosening up my menu plan, I realized I was moving from weight-loss mode into maintenance mode in a natural and easy fashion. This thought thrilled me, because in the past I have been very much an on- or-off-the diet person, which is why I yo-yoed a lot.

At first I was strict seven days a week, then I moved into weight-loss mode on weekdays and maintenance on weekends. This was still not a free-for-all though. I was not going back to snacking and choosing the junky foods that had been my downfall in the past.

I still stuck to three meals a day, but I was a bit more easy-going within those meals. I also still stuck to 'no sugar', but I returned to enjoying a bliss ball paired with a piece of ninety-percent-cacao chocolate after dinner. If we ate out, I enjoyed every bit of my meal, but I didn't order dessert. After we arrived home I wrote in the notebook the name of the dish I had and the restaurant we had eaten at.

Don't quit your success practices too soon

I felt like my notebook method was helping a lot with consistency, but once I began writing down the same meals and portion sizes day after day I wondered if I should not bother writing everything down.

After musing out loud to my husband, he made a good point. He thought it was a good idea to continue writing down my meals, weight, days etc., because it was all part of the process. This was after a relatively short time that I thought about quitting the notebook too; because even though I wasn't at my goal weight, I felt like I was in a good routine.

I decided to continue with my notebook – I still had many pages left in it – and my genius touch to keep me enthused right through to my goal weight and beyond, was to write my goal weight on the very last page at the back of the notebook.

Now whenever I feel like my meals have all become a bit routine, I look at the last page and remember what I want. I would highly recommend this little tip. I'd like to note that my goal weight is not too low either. I am not one of those women who want to be artificially thin;

to be honest I don't think I'd be able to do that because I like food too much.

Setting a goal weight

How I worked out my goal weight was from an old-fashioned formula I read about in a vintage etiquette book. The advice said that a woman should be one hundred pounds for the first five feet of her height, with an extra five pounds for every inch.

I love to read advice like this from another era, so I worked out for my five-foot-seven height, that my weight by this method should be 135 pounds, which is around 61kg. When I was a Weight Watchers member many years ago, I remember that the weight range for my height was 58kg-72kg (for both women and men).

I am not trying to be skinnier than is healthy and feel that 61kg is a reasonable weight to aim for. I am not fixated on this weight either, it is simply a number I have set. If I get down to 65kg or 63kg and feel happy with how I look and feel, I will happily stop there.

Having the notebook right there on the kitchen counter means it is easy to jot down my meals as I go through my day – sometimes before, sometimes after. It is a simple system and I think that's why I have stuck with it for so long.

Committing myself to a daily practice means I am also committing myself to doing what it takes, every day. It keeps me focused on my goal.

Your *Thirty Slim Days* action tips:

Start a dedicated notebook for your journey to slim. Even if you are part way through your weight loss already, a daily account will help you continue.

Head up the page each day with:

The date
What day it is in your notebook (Day 1, Day 2, etc.)
Your weight if you have weighed yourself
Your period days if you have them (P1, P2, etc.)
>   *(this helped me not be freaked out by a higher weight at different times of the month)*

And **write your goal weight on the last page**. I am excited looking forward to the time I get to that last page; filling in one each day, I will *be* that weight. I don't mind saying that I am not there yet, but I am closer than I have ever been in consistency of practice and days without junky food binges. I already feel like I am there in my mind, and my body is catching up in its own time.

I haven't counted the pages to see how many days it will be until my goal weight; because I want to keep it as a surprise plus I don't want to put pressure on myself.

If you don't feel comfortable with being as open as I am about your slimming notebook, keep it closed or in a more private place. I would recommend you be as transparent as possible though.

Hopefully those you live with want the best for you and are willing to be your cheerleaders. **Enlist their support** and in due course you will find yourself writing in the last page of your notebook, celebrating your goal weight.

Day 4
Why do you want to be slim?

What if I asked you the question *Why do you want to be slim?* What would you say to that? You might think I am being funny, because, well, isn't it obvious?

There will be answers that come to mind straight away. But if that was the case, why are you not there already? I always wanted be a consistently lower weight and feel peaceful around food, but I was neither. Why? What was stopping me?

Taking the time to dig a little deeper and come up with a compelling list of reasons that you can refer to at times when you are tempted to give up is a fantastic mood lifter to have. Consider all aspects of your life: your health and comfort, family, job, money, home life, everything.

To succeed with a goal, you must have a big 'why'. It isn't enough of a motivator to simply have a goal with no purpose, and only a few superficial reasons; or even worse – because you 'should'. You will not stay the path to achieve your goal without excellent reasons to get you past the initial enthusiasm of starting another diet.

When I asked myself the question '**Why do I want to lose weight?**', I came up with:

- To have a strong and healthy body
- To be slim and look good
- To enjoy my fashionable wardrobe
- To feel good physically and mentally
- To have a glowing complexion
- To feel happy and well every day
- To live as long as I can in as good a health as I can
- To give myself the best chance of a long and healthy life
- To enjoy my life now and when I am older too
- To feel sexy for myself and my husband
- To enjoy the everyday
- To save money – not buying junk food, not wasting clothes I can't fit
- To feel good about myself
- To have higher self-esteem
- To not feel self-conscious
- To be able to wear anything and have it look good on me

- To feel like I have conquered this problem area of my life
- To not be beholden to unhealthy foods and habits
- To feel physically comfortable in my clothes

If I really wanted all these things – and I do! I've wanted them for years – why was I not there yet? Why was I still setting the same weight goals year after year and never quite reaching them?

So I asked myself:

What kinds of things do I do to sabotage that? What is stopping me from achieving a healthy body?

- I give in to cravings and eat sugar
- I don't plan ahead, so there is often not a healthy meal organized
- I think *What's the point? I'm always going to be this size so I may as well enjoy myself*
- I focus on what I can't have i.e. junk food, instead of what I want i.e. a healthy, happy body
- I am eating bigger portions than I need
- I don't like to feel hunger – I get jittery – so I eat to soothe that feeling
- I love to eat foods that taste good to me, no matter their quality
- I don't like to feel deprived

- I feel like I am missing out – others have it, why can't I?
- I want to have fun – life is so dreary without treats

All the unhealthy and sabotaging habits we have, they are giving us something or we wouldn't do them. Addressing the benefits of the way we currently eat and then working out ways to get those benefits in other ways will also help us towards our goal.

That's why we can feel like we are being deprived or having our favourite foods 'taken away from us' when we start a diet. Is it any wonder we rebel and start eating all the foods we swore we'd never eat again?

Our subconscious mind loves comfort and the status quo. It loves for everything *to be the same, forever* because it's comfortable that way. It knows what is going to come next and there is no effort required on its part.

When we start laying down the law and saying, *I'm only going to eat three strict paleo meals per day, no snacks; drinks and nibbles only on a Saturday night*, what do you think we are thinking deep-down? To get the best idea, perhaps picture a two-year old that you've taken their favourite toy from, giving them an educational learning set in return...

Let's look at the benefits I gain from my unhealthy eating habits.

What benefits do I gain from eating the way I have in the past?

For me, I would say:

- It's fun to eat whatever I want
- I love sweet foods and I love to indulge in them
- It's time-out for me with the sofa, something to read and a bowl of potato chips
- I feel happy when I am eating chocolate
- It brings back good family memories to eat treat foods (birthday parties, Christmas, Easter eggs etc.)
- I am giving love to myself
- I am treating myself
- I don't like to miss out (FOMO!)
- It tastes good

There is a flipside to those benefits though. If there wasn't, I would have been happy, healthy and slim already, and likely not writing this book.

There are always consequences to any action we do, whether they are good or bad consequences. With eating, we tend to blank out on the consequences, instead preferring to focus on how good the food tastes. But what are we depriving ourselves of by eating as we do?

Here's my list:

What am I missing out on by eating the way I have done in the past?

- Feeling good about myself
- Looking nice in my clothes
- Fitting some of my clothes – some jeans it's been years since I've worn them
- Sleeping well – if I've been eating sugar I sleep terribly
- Feeling like a success
- Feeling worthy
- Having better health
- Not feeling self-conscious about my food choices and my weight

If we try to put ourselves on a strict diet and don't address our mindset, it might start out easy with the novelty of a new and exciting plan, but at some stage the novelty will wear off and our inner two-year-old will not want to play along any more – there *will* be tantrums.

It's much easier to address that before it happens and put measures in place that will mean we are happy to carry on with our new healthy way of living. We will want to find other ways to get benefits we have gained from eating the way we have in the past – healthier ways.

We already have our list of benefits, so it's a matter of going through that list and brainstorming other ways to get the desired rewards; or, reframing the way we think about the perceived payoffs.

For me:

How can I reframe healthy eating from deprivation to my preferred option?

- It's more fun to feel slender and vibrant than to eat junk
- I will be honouring the woman I want to be
- I will be slimmer, no doubt
- I will feel peaceful instead of tortured
- Peppermint tea is much more chic than kiddie lollies in a family-size bag
- I won't cause my skin to age quicker with all that sugar in my system
- I won't give myself type-two diabetes or any other blood-sugar related illness
- I will feel proud
- I will feel like a grown-up
- I will save money
- I won't be known by my family as the one with a sweet tooth
- I won't feel like such an addict from craving sugar
- I know it will be easier once it's a habit and then I won't even think about snacking

- My clothes will fit beautifully
- Everything I wear will looking amazing on me

Recreating the benefits of snacking is easy. I can create a list of enticing non-food activities such as reading my current book, taking a nap, watching an episode of my favourite television program, starting or continuing a craft project – basically giving myself *time* for all the pastimes I enjoy.

That's what I realized all my sofa nibbling was about – I was wanting to take a break but felt guilty about it, so I created a craving for a snack that meant I had to sit down and rest. After all, I couldn't very well clean the bathroom while having a snack.

Now let's think about all the benefits of getting into a routine of healthy meals with less processed junk food.

How will I gain from eating healthier on a consistent basis?

- I will feel peaceful around food and eating, and more peaceful in general
- I will feel balanced and in control
- I will feel proud of myself
- I will have no guilt or regret like I do when I gorge myself on candy/chocolate/ice-cream
- I will feel physically comfortable
- I will feel happy with myself
- I will feel strong and capable

- I will feel good about myself (increased self-esteem/self-worth)
- I won't get as many headaches/migraines
- I will save money, both on junky foods and also buying headache pills every so often
- I will be healthier
- I will have clearer thinking
- I will be showing my body respect and compassion
- I will be looking after my body
- I will have healthy cells and an improved immune system
- I won't be thinking about food all the time
- I will feel vibrant and energetic
- I will feel more youthful – I am slowing down the aging process
- I will sleep well
- I will feel sexier

I don't know about you, but I find this list extremely motivating. Sometimes it is literally a thought that can make me go one way or the other, so having the above reasons in mind could be the difference between buying and eating something crappy... or not. And the less I do it, the stronger the habit of not eating junk gets. Conversely, the more I give in, the stronger the habit of eating junk gets.

I love writing motivating ideas for myself; here are a few more that I enjoyed the results of:

My main goal is to enjoy a peaceful relationship with food. Why do I want this?

- It will be more relaxing
- I won't have to worry about overdoing it and putting on weight
- I will see food as my friend
- It will remove the drama around food for me
- It will be easier to decide what to eat and not eat
- It will be simpler to have three meals a day and not snack on junk
- It sounds as if how normal people feel about food
- It will take the power away from certain junky foods
- It will put food back in its rightful place as enjoyable nourishment
- I will no longer obsess over certain foods
- I will feel better about myself
- My weight will normalize over time without me having to work for it

And:

What can I do to have a healthy body?

- Sleep well and for enough time

- Drink water all day
- Eat healthy, fresh foods that nourish me
- Go easy on foods that leave me feeling bogged down – have them less often
- Have regular health checks
- Exercise every day
- Promote positive thoughts
- Surround myself with beauty, love and happiness
- Find hobbies I enjoy to replace snacking

I know there are *a lot* of lists in this chapter, but I wanted to show you that you can create your own personalized inspiration by going within and asking yourself 'What do I want?'

We spend so much time reading others points of view on how best to feed and look ourselves, but have you ever really stopped to think 'What would feel best to ME?' Ask yourself in a loving way 'What would I like?', 'What do you want to tell me?' When I've done this, I've had the most random but *inspired* answers pop into my head.

It's the magic of the mind and you have all the answers inside you too. It's great to read information about a topic you are interested in; I love all the Kindle books I have downloaded; *and* it's wonderful to set everything aside at least once a day and ask yourself 'What do I want to do today?'

It feels totally decadent!

Your *Thirty Slim Days* action tips:

Ask yourself the following questions; try for at least five answers per question, preferably ten or even twenty. Set yourself a number and your mind will comply. There is no need to answer them all at once; pick one that looks appealing and go from there.

Why do I want to be slimmer?

What do I do to sabotage that? What is stopping me from achieving a healthy body?

What benefits do I gain from eating the way I have in the past?

What am I missing out on by eating the way I have done in the past?

How can I recreate those benefits in other ways?

How can I reframe healthy eating from deprivation to my preferred option?

How will I gain from eating healthier on a consistent basis?

What do I want to feel like on a daily basis when it comes to food and my body?

How can I create that for myself?

Going through these questions and writing down answers for yourself helps your mind get on board with your wishes. You are **cajoling and coaxing** yourself along, rather than shouting at yourself like an army major. Not only does it feel nicer, but it works much better too.

Day 5
The chic kitchen

Whenever I feel a bit bogged down and am not eating as well as I'd like, what always helps is to fine-tune my kitchen. It's fairly clutter-free from previous go-overs, but whenever I do revisit it, I find clutter that has crept back in.

I am a big fan of Peter Walsh's books. I've read them all, plus have most of them as audiobooks, so I can brainwash myself when I am out walking or doing the housework. One of his books is called '*Does this clutter make my butt look fat?*' and it's about the link between the excess weight on our body and the excess clutter in our home, particularly the kitchen.

In my kitchen, utensils, pots and dishes are under control from previous declutterings, but the pantry is a different story. It is not a great design to start with: the shelves are deep and the opening is small. It doesn't take much to start looking too full; food gets pushed to the back and I forget about items I have bought.

Every so often when the messiness builds up, I remove all foodstuffs from the pantry and put it on the kitchen counter. The shelves get a quick wipe-down and then I put everything back. I don't usually have to throw anything out since I do the pantry shuffle on regular basis, but I do pull forward ingredients I want to use up before they expire.

Even though the same number of items have gone back into the pantry, it feels very different. I can see everything at once and order is restored. I stage it to look stylish and it looks so nice. Plastic storage baskets group together items and this keeps my pantry tidier for longer.

Imagining one of my elegant lady-friends peeking into the pantry gives me extra enthusiasm. What if my poodle friend Barbara saw how messy and untidy everything was when her home is so lovely. What if Lauren from Instagram with the enticingly organized home saw the mess of my shelves? These thoughts are great motivation when I am tidying and beautifying my kitchen.

Treat your kitchen as if it was your dream kitchen

Our kitchen is not new or fancy, but it looks far better when it is clean and tidy than otherwise. When we first moved into our 1990-built house, I couldn't wait for the day when we had a sparkling new, beautiful kitchen.

Five years later, we still have the original kitchen. We decided to put the money into paying off our home loan quicker instead and now that we are debt-free, I am more than happy with our decision.

But I don't see why I shouldn't have an inspiring kitchen space right now. A space that motivates me to create healthy and nourishing meals to keep my body happy and trim.

I love browsing homes for sale online, and find staged homes very motivating. They look so magazine-like and inviting. I love the way staged kitchens have nothing on the counter apart from one or two items. This is my goal when I declutter, organize and clean our kitchen.

Being a place that is used many times a day to prepare meals and hot drinks, it is no wonder items migrate around and get jammed in the same old place even if that place is already full. Products that are used frequently are also left out which adds to a messy, non-magazine look and that is not the visual I am after.

Our kitchen is twenty-seven-years-old, but I still want it to look stylishly simple, and I love to keep it clean and organized. If it was all new and wonderful that would be amazing of course, but I truly am just as happy with it as it is right now.

Don't wait for the day when you have a new kitchen. Treat your kitchen today as if it was royalty.

For me, I find this approach helps me stay slim, because I am in touch with the food we have available; and the tidiness helps me be motivated to put together a delicious and healthy meal.

When your kitchen is cluttered, untidy and dirty it is so much easier to pick up unhealthy fast food or decide to eat out. A messy kitchen is not an attractive place to be, so it's no surprise if you don't want to spend time in it.

How to overcome mindless nibbling and boredom or procrastination hunger when at home

You may find this quite revolutionary (I did, even though it was the most obvious solution around): don't have your problem foods in the pantry. Keep them *at the shop*, where it's much less handy to eat them. Yes, you still have the option to go and get them, but the convenience barrier is there.

When I have told myself, *You can have whatever snacks you want, Fiona, but you have to go out and get them*, it stopped me most of the time. The rare time I'd go; but mostly I couldn't be bothered driving to the supermarket for a packet of chips or a bar or chocolate, so I'd go without or have something else instead.

It wasn't only the inconvenience either. If I felt like potato chips late in the afternoon (a recurring theme for me back in the day), I'd then think of the long queues of people at the checkout getting their dinner groceries after work.

And if I felt like chocolate or ice-cream after dinner, I'd picture the strange rag-tag bunch of people who cruise supermarket aisles at night. I know because I've been one of them.

You might be one of those organized people who grocery shop at off-times such as 9pm on a Wednesday and there are always one or two of those, but mostly it is ghostly-looking apparitions floating down the junk food aisles seeing what they feel like. I didn't like being associated with that. It was honestly like junkies looking for their fix!

Once I got it into my head that all the weirdos came out at night, I didn't want to go then either. I am easily spooked and the weirdo factor cured my after-dinner snacking habit.

Don't be tempted by super-specials to stock up on your favourite snacking foods either. Even though I mostly did the 'keep my favourite snacks at the store' technique, I could still have my head turned by a 4/$5 bargain. *Ooh that's cheap*, I'd tell myself. I'd buy them, eat lots over the week, feel revolting and then remember – yet again – why I used my inconvenience technique.

Instead, keep fresh fruit, bliss balls, almonds, nice tea bags or coffee and chilled sparkling mineral water to hand. You are far more likely to eat what is there simply by the proximity factor.

Detach yourself from your groceries

It can be easier to advise or shop for someone else, so detach yourself from your shopping trolley and pretend you are picking up goodies for a dear friend who is laid up in bed after a foot operation. You wouldn't take her jumbo bags of cheese-flavoured corn snacks because they are cheap, would you?

If it was me I would take a few ripe peaches or whatever fruit was in season, a box of gourmet crackers and a wedge of brie, a jar of olives, pyramid tea-bags and a bar of 90% cacao swiss chocolate. Very nice.

What about shopping as if you were stocking the fridge for Euro-royals on their yacht? What might they like? Think healthy, delicious and refined.

Setting yourself up for success is all about making your kitchen an elegant and welcoming place to be. You have decluttered items that you don't use, cleaned up your pantry and fridge and vowed to leave ugly snack foods at the store, replacing them with elegant options instead.

Find creative new ideas to try

The next step is to harness your creativity which has been unleashed by your streamlined and reorganized kitchen and make healthy food exciting, not worthy. I always feel inspired to eat different foods and present my meals in more creative ways when I have spent time reorganizing our kitchen. It is a petite version of how a trip away shakes up your inner world and inspires you to try new experiences.

When we were busy in our business we would find ourselves stuck in a rut with meals, simply because we had no time to think of anything new. Now that we have sold our business and are in limbo for a short time before we move to the small town where we plan to live, I find we are eating differently – healthier and more creatively.

Yesterday my husband and I did some errands in town and had a quick salad out too. We then decided to stop off at a beach-side café on the way home for a coffee. It was such a pleasant half-hour and at little cost too, since we don't often buy coffees out.

The café we were at also did full meals and I happened to glance up at the specials board and saw a dukkah-crusted fish menu item with delicious sounding Mediterranean vegetables. 'That looks nice for a dinner idea', I commented to my husband (probably not what the café intended when they chalked up the menu).

'Let's have it tonight', he said. So we stopped in at the grocery store on our way home and picked up fresh snapper white-fish and a bag of yummy looking gourmet spiced dukkah. Our inspired meal was beautiful with oven-baked dukkah-crusted snapper and multitudes of brightly-coloured vegetables.

'I think that's the first time I have ever offered to have fish for dinner' he said, because usually my husband looks at fish as the healthy option that never fills him up. And it was all because of a chance sighting at a café when we were doing something out of our normal routine.

Do you need any new equipment?

Another way to set yourself up for success is to get kitchen items that you need. If you find yourself constantly thinking 'that would be good', why not look into it. Two items that I purchased and have used a lot already are a spiralizer, and a pair of salad lunchboxes.

Because we are eating less pasta, I wanted to try a spiralizer. I didn't want to spend a lot in case I didn't end up using it as much as I imagined, but neither did I want to buy a cheap piece of junk. I found an Oxo spiralizer that fit right in the middle. It is fun to use for salads and I have also made spaghetti bolognaise with zoodles (zucchini noodles). In New Zealand we also call this vegetable courgette, so the alternative name we came up with was courgoodles (with a soft 'g'). Such fun! The Oxo spiralizer is sturdy and easy to clean. Perfect.

With the lunchboxes, I was making salads to take to work each day and once we had sold the shop but still needed to spend the next month there training the new staff, there was suddenly no fridge available. I found inexpensive Sistema salad containers with a little icepack that slots into the lid so you don't need a fridge to keep your salad chilled.

Little did I know that the lunchboxes would instantly make our salads more enjoyable. I can't believe how easily influenced I am by packaging sometimes. The lunchboxes came with their own knife and fork and a tiny dressing bottle. It was fun to make them at night, almost like I was making salads for someone else, and then when it came to lunchtime the next day I had a ready-made meal as if I'd bought it from a gourmet café.

When we had a fridge at work I would keep vegetables there and chop them at the time. I quickly found that a pre-prepared salad tests your willpower much less when you are hungry and there are multiple takeaway options right outside your door.

We have also used our salad containers for a quick and healthy road-trip lunch, day-trips to the beach on the weekend and a spot of relaxing at beautiful Cornwall Park, a large public area here in Auckland.

Create healthy versions of your favourite foods

Making healthy food something to look forward to is key to your success when it comes to becoming and staying slim. Come up with meals that excite you so that your old favourites won't tempt you as much.

Along the same lines, revolutionize your favourite unhealthy meals by coming up with your own versions to cook at home. This isn't a new idea and you will find many recipes online if you search for your own favourite. I remember seeing recipes for homemade

KFC coating many years ago and being quite excited by that!

For us, we recreate fish and chips, Chili's dinners of chicken tenders, baked potato and coleslaw, thin-crust pizza, nachos with corn chips and more. It might be a bit fiddly the first time, but once you've cooked it, it will be easier each time after that. You can tweak it to suit your family's palette each time.

My husband loves a Big Mac but doesn't often have one because he wants to be healthy. Sometimes we will have homemade hamburgers and chips made from scratch which are delicious, but the day he found a familiar-coloured 'burger sauce' at the supermarket that he said tastes exactly like Big Mac Sauce, I think that made him a very happy man!

Now perhaps recreating takeaway meals doesn't equate to a chic kitchen for you, but I am a realist. As much as I would love to be chic and refined one-hundred-percent of the time, I do like something a bit more casual every now and then.

And that's what I am all about – being inspired by an elevated way of being, but not hemming myself into a chic yet constricting box. Being a better version of myself still includes being myself.

It's a fine line, but I think we all know when we are kidding ourselves. Are we eating healthy most of the time with only once-in-a-while forays onto the unchic side of the road? If so, those meals are a vital and necessary part of living a life with spice – that touch of kitsch that the French woman does so well.

Your *Thirty Slim Days* action tips:

Look at your kitchen with fresh eyes. Don't see how old it is or how shabby everything looks; rather, look at how it could be improved at no cost.

Is every cupboard decluttered, neat and tidy, with items ready to use easily?
Is it free of junky foodstuffs?
What about your fridge and freezer – are there mystery foods that need to go?

Spend a little time **creating your own chic kitchen**, asking yourself if the elegant dream version of you would have *this* in her pantry. You don't have to do everything at once – you can start with one cupboard and do a little at a time.

Wipe shelves down and clean doors inside and out as you go and I promise you will have a new appreciation for your kitchen, old or not.

Clean out junky foods. Remove any unchic snack foods and either put them in one cupboard, or even better, in another room. The times when I did buy multiples of snack foods because they were on a super-special, I kept them in a supermarket bag in the closet of the guest room.

They were out of sight, which also kept them out of my stomach. Until I ate them of course, but I ate them less because they weren't right in front of me every time

I opened the pantry door. Now, I don't buy them at all, but keeping them in another place is a good first step.

If you must buy snack foods for others, buy flavours and items that you don't like, but they do. I have used this technique successfully in the past. Someone I lived with preferred chicken-flavoured potato chips which could never tempt me, thank goodness. I happily bought them each week and never ate one, no willpower necessary.

Shop as if you were being paid to by an elegant and slender lady. This can be a fun way to avoid impulse purchases of unstylish snack foods. You will want to choose foods that please her. If you can spend a little bit, make her a wealthy, elegant and slender lady. If you are on a strict budget, pretend she has given you a tiny amount that you must make go as far as possible while still being healthy and filling.

You are that elegant and slender lady. You deserve good, real foods that nourish you, not cheap junk. You are worth more than that. You have what it takes to feed yourself in a healthy and delicious way. You know you do.

Day 6
Living a life of alignment

Is feeling aligned to your dream life a key to becoming and staying slender?

I have been exploring this fascinating concept for a while now, and it comes down to this:

If you are not living a life in alignment with your true wishes and desires; if you are not fulfilling the purpose of why you are here, this could be one of the reasons why you overeat.

- *You overeat to gain control when you feel you have no control over a situation.*
- *You overeat to feel pleasure in a life filled with obligations seemingly not of your choosing.*
- *You overeat to rebel against others expectations of you (the 'You can't control me' thought)*

- *You comfort eat to do something pleasurable for yourself*

When you are engaged in activities you enjoy, you have less need for excess food. When you feel more in control of how you live your life, the need for comfort food falls away.

For sixteen years I worked at various office jobs – Personal Assistant, Executive Assistant, Secretary, Office Manager, Office Administrator, etc.

Even though I thought these were the types of jobs I was good at and could enjoy, I was bored to tears typing up letters and reports and came to hate leaving the house each day. That sounds pretty dramatic and it wasn't as bad as that; and yes, I do know that no-one goes to work for fun and some have far worse jobs than I did.

But what I really wanted was to be at home. I loved being in my own surroundings, having my own timeframe, seeing my pets, pottering, even enjoying doing my housework because I had the time.

Going to my job was a necessity of course, because I liked earning money to pay the rent and buy groceries. When I bought lunch at work, I'd also buy a bag of something fun to make my afternoon a little brighter – candy I could nibble on throughout the afternoon. That daily habit was the sunshine of my day and naturally it made me stack on the weight.

It became a bit better when my husband and I started our own business. Working in retail meant I was up and down from my desk with customers, and I did not become so bored.

There were still days when I'd disappear across the road to buy a bag of sweet treats for myself though. I needed a bit of levity from the paperwork and supplier issues not to mention the 'fun' that sometimes comes with dealing with the public.

I still craved to spend my days at home. I enjoyed my retail work at the time, the nice customers anyway; but as an introvert I found my energy was severely depleted by all that people contact.

Now that I am entering my new phase of working from home as a writer, I feel fortunate that I don't need to fight the traffic to go to a workplace each day. Others might not mind that and I know people who love to get out of the house and be somewhere else surrounded by people; but for me, being at home is a fabulous feeling.

Already I can feel the peace and calm that is coming from being where I want to be. It's not the perfect mirage I thought it might be; I am still working out a daily schedule and finding how to self-motivate now that I don't have external pressures, but I couldn't be happier.

How is my afternoon sweet treat habit going, you ask? I don't need to nibble on candy anymore and a big part of it is down to living my life in alignment with my dreams.

What do you dream of doing?

A great question to ask yourself is: If you could do any job, anywhere; what would it be? If training, skills, money and family obligations were no consideration, what would you love to do with your life?

Don't worry if your dreams are so big you think they are ridiculous. Don't listen to the voice in your head that says you are too young, too old, live in the wrong place or any other silly reason.

If it's a new career, can you take steps towards it? Can you do something related to it as a side job? Can you take it up as an unpaid hobby to start with and see what happens?

This is how writing started for me. From a young age I have loved reading and I read a lot of books. In addition, I have always dreamed of writing a book. So, I started a blog, plus I began writing chapters towards my book. I tried fiction and it didn't feel like me, even though I always imagined myself writing a fiction book. It ended up that non-fiction, for now anyway, is where my flow is. I find it fun and easy to write non-fiction and it's almost like I am speaking through my fingers.

From writing my blog posts, I tested self-publishing by compiling favourite posts into small Kindle books. People ordered them! That was a revelation to me and gave me the confidence to continue with my long-neglected non-fiction book that had been coming along behind the scenes.

It had been outlined and partially written for a number of years. One day, I realized that the only way it was going to be written was for me to write it. Writing it wasn't the problem though, self-belief was. I'd write a bit and think 'that's dumb' and put it away for another six months. I'd find it again and read a bit. 'It's really good!' I'd tell myself. So I'd write a bit more and then talk myself down again.

Finally I made myself finish it. I mentioned on my blog that I was doing it to give myself public accountability, and a dear blog reader offered to edit for me. I had involved other people now, so I had to finish it. Then, once it was finished and published, I was on a roll. All my other books that had been backing up could be set free, and they are, with many more to come.

For you, do you want to be a writer? Perhaps you dream of selling your sewing, knitting or needlework on Etsy. My sister did that. She went from being a complete beginner, learning how to sew when she had her first baby.

She started making baby clothes and selling them on Etsy to create a part-time income for herself, plus she had a creative outlet. A decade on and her pattern-drafting and dressmaking skills are out-of-sight good.

There is surely a skill that you have that you love to do, that you can turn into your career, enjoy on the side as a source of part-time income or have as a very satisfying hobby. These days there are very few businesses that cannot be monetized online and there has never been a better time in history to go after your dreams.

You don't have to quit your job

Perhaps you don't particularly desire to be an entrepreneur and work for yourself; you are more than happy to have a job to go to and earn a living without having to think about it too much.

Is that job right for you though? Looking back at my office 'career', I might have been better in a sales environment. When I worked in our retail business, I found that I was naturally good at sales, in a soft-sell kind of way.

I enjoyed getting to know the customers and had a high strike-rate simply from talking to them in a way that I would want to be spoken to. I remembered them when they came in again and followed up when I said I would. Customers brought me in cake and gifts at Christmas and would specifically visit on the days I worked sometimes. Some have even become friends.

If I had my time again, likely I would have become a writer much sooner, but if I had to apply for a job I would have looked in the sales section of the newspaper rather than the office roles I automatically looked to.

Living a life of alignment is not only about your job, although employment is a huge component. Consider every aspect of your life and ask yourself if it's what you really want.

What hobbies and pastimes could you enjoy?

With your downtime at home, think about all the fun pastimes you could enjoy instead of snacking. For me, it's crafty pursuits because I love knitting, sewing, patchwork, crochet and needlepoint. I also love to read, go for walks listening to podcasts and audiobooks, organize and declutter our home and write.

If you say 'I have no downtime, Fiona', perhaps that's the problem. Having no time for hobbies and pastimes that you enjoy sounds like it could be a prime reason to overeat – for pleasure and as time-out for yourself.

Surely you can schedule in one or two hours a week where you do exactly as you please – visit the gallery for a spot of art appreciation, sign up for a wine tasting course, or start a craft or writing project that you work on each Sunday afternoon. There are so many ways to explore your passions, and when you do so, eating is not your only pleasure or escape.

It is highly likely that weight loss will be a side benefit of living a fulfilled and creative life where we focus on the activities that we want and desire to do, rather than trying not to eat the wrong foods.

When we are enjoying ourselves pottering around with a hobby; maybe painting a watercolour or sketching in a notebook, we can enter a state of flow where we don't notice time passing. Being in this state is very calming and satisfying, almost meditative.

If we pursue weight loss as its own goal, it seems to elude us. But if we engage in activities that bring us happiness and satisfaction – activities that engage creativity in our brain – it takes the focus off weight loss, food and eating. This is healthy not only for your body, but your mind as well.

Your *Thirty Slim Days* action tips:

What were those **dreams you had as a child** that you packed away and have not thought about for a long time? Think of the activities you loved the most and bring them out to play with.

What kind of work would you be doing if you asked yourself 'what job or career would I love to have?'

Make a list of all the **fun activities** you would enjoy doing and choose one to spend time on this week.

If you have to leave the house by yourself to ensure you follow through, then do that.

- Take your laptop or a notebook to start your book and write at a beautiful five-star hotel café for an hour.
- Take your book or handcraft project to the park and spread out a rug, sunning your legs with big sunglasses on.

- Bundle up and take the subway into the city to wander around photographing the architecture.

Don't stop believing!

Believe that you deserve to **live a life of fun and happiness**. You might believe that you must slog your way to retirement, but it's not true. Start living your life in alignment *today* by doing what you enjoy and not settling for a second-class life.

You, my friend, are first-class all the way.

Day 7
Keep your frequency high

Everything you want in life is usually desired because it will make you feel good. It is human instinct that we will look to fulfil our need to feel good on a regular basis, whether we realize it or not.

At its simplest, keeping your frequency high is simply about creating that good feeling. Or to put it another way – you will know that your frequency is high because you feel good.

When you are in an increased frequency you have new thoughts; more powerful thoughts where you can then create your reality. You draw different experiences to you depending on whether your frequency is higher or lower.

Making a regular choice to keep yourself in a high frequency as much as possible, whether it's the clothes you wear or the environment you are in will affect how successful you are in your life and with your eating habits.

When you are in a high frequency it is a breeze to prepare healthy and delicious foods, be well-groomed, dress in a way that inspires you and be an all-round happy person for yourself and others.

There are many ways to raise your frequency, and it's a two-way street: you find it easier to eat well when you are feeling good, but you can also make yourself feel good by eating nourishing, colourful food.

You feel like making the effort with your appearance when you're feeling good, but you can also make yourself feel good by taking an extra five or ten minutes to put on some makeup, do your hair and choose a nice outfit when you get ready in the morning.

Speak yourself happy

I love to use mantras and sayings to help keep me in a good frequency. The quote *'Today I will do what others won't – so tomorrow I can do what others can't'* is a favourite. It reminds me that it's okay to be different to everyone else.

Sure, I may be quizzed about my food choices because I don't want a slice of cake with my afternoon coffee, but that's okay. I am eating today what others won't, so I can be as slim and healthy as I like tomorrow. I am willing to ignore advertising and what everyone else is eating today, so that I can have a body like no-one else's tomorrow.

And that's the truth. The truth is that most people aren't prepared to put time and effort into their health. They aren't prepared to shop for fresh produce and healthy food items and spend time preparing them.

They would rather look at highly-promoted advertising to tell them what to eat. They would rather satisfy their every whim, even if it leads to poor health and a body that looks and feels unattractive.

I know, because I have been that person. I have eaten my favourite snack foods every day and thought I was having fun, but my unhappiness and low frequency told another story.

With our western world surroundings, it's a lot harder than in other more traditional countries to eat healthy and be slim. We are starting off on the back foot. That's why it is so important to keep a high frequency as much as possible, to be able to avoid the temptations that are thrown in our face, literally around every corner.

Be clean, be serene

Another way of keeping my frequency high is to stay organized, tidy and clean. When I let areas become messy and dirty because I've been too busy or unmotivated to address them, I notice it affects other parts of my life. I become less discriminating with what I put into my mouth. Treat foods sneak their way back into the pantry.

The messiness is lowering my frequency and I am looking for a way to feel better – by snacking.

It's harder to become motivated about cleaning than it is to sit down with a book and a sweet treat, yes, I completely agree. But I found that when I started with just one area, I felt better. The sugar craving wasn't so strong and my housework didn't seem so insurmountable. I didn't need to make the whole house show-home-perfect; I only needed to start with one area. Then another, and another.

I recently tidied my writing desk which has my computer, pens, paper, journals and a printer on it. Since we sold our business and had moved all our paperwork to our home office, I didn't have any new systems set up. There was no-where for the bills to land, so they stayed on the corner of my writing desk.

I didn't want to interrupt my writing to do filing and account reconciling, so I left it to one side to do once a week (which did not happen). As the pile grew, it attracted other items and soon my desk looked and felt horrible. I couldn't dust it because of all the items on it, so there were cat hairs and dust bunnies as well.

I thought to myself 'I don't have time to clean up, I want to finish writing this book and then I'll do it. I knew this was going about it the wrong way though; if I wanted to feel motivated to write I needed a clean and tidy workspace. So I took everything off my desk apart from the big items, placing them on the floor in piles.

I dusted my desk and computer equipment before filing papers, finding new homes for everything and working as quickly as possible until everything was off the floor and either put away, dealt with or thrown out.

It took me about half a day and was time well spent. My productivity went through the roof as my creativity was unstifled. Afterwards I also realized I had started eating at my desk – because of the mess!

When I first set my office area up I told myself it was a food-free zone. A cup of tea or glass of water was fine, but no food. I wasn't going to sit there on the computer day after day getting fatter from all the nibbling, plus having one of those icky keyboards that is full of crumbs.

But not long before I cleaned my desk up, I bought a packet of Snowballs – marshmallow pieces covered in chocolate and rolled in coconut. I stuffed my face with them one day *at my desk*. It wasn't my finest moment; normally I saved my snacking for the sofa.

When I moved my keyboard to clean my desk, all the little pieces of coconut reminded me of that day, when my frequency was perilously low. And it was all caused by the messiness of my desk! Thankfully the cycle was broken, and now I wouldn't dream of bringing food into my office (even healthy food).

Affirm yourself into the woman you want to be

Talking yourself up is a great vibration lifter too. If you find yourself stuck in a funk or a downward spiral where you think *you'll never get this weight thing under control*, be your own cheerleader.

I find affirmations fabulous for this. There are many you can find around – simply google 'weight loss affirmations', but I find creating my own really hits the spot. You can think about how your ideal self would be, re-write negative thoughts as their positive opposite and list attributes of successfully slim people as if it were you talking.

Here are some of my favourites. I added to this list over time, and I read it often. Some days I'll read it morning, noon and night if I need to.

I am a chic success.
I am in control of everything I think.
I am in control of everything I eat.
I love making being slim and healthy fun
I have the same motivation no matter what I weigh
I forgive myself for eating as I have in the past; I am
*   different now*
I choose to have smaller portions and feel happy
*   about it*
It is okay for me to have three healthy meals a day
*   without snacking*
I have chosen to eliminate refined sugar from my diet
I prefer to feel a little bit hungry before meals
It is okay for me to eat different foods than others if I
*   choose to*
I make my own food decisions
It is okay for me to say 'no thank you'

I am learning to deeply and completely love and accept my body

I find it easy to be consistent with healthy eating because I remind myself that I love being slim and healthy

My weight has dropped without effort to the perfect level for me

I sleep 8-9 hours every night and love going to bed early

I am learning to be more consistent with my eating and weight

I find it easy to be consistent with my positive slimming thoughts

I adore my slim physique

I am so happy and grateful that I can wear all my gorgeous outfits and they all look amazing

I love being inspired to be slim and stylish like the girls in The Devil Wears Prada movie

My wardrobe is edited and curated and reflects me perfectly – slimming down my wardrobe made it easy for me to slim down my body

Decluttering and keeping our home clutter-free helps me stay slim

Prioritizing my jobs and doing the most important tasks first helps me stay slim

I love to feel light by eating light foods

I find it easy to think up interesting, healthy and easy meals

I love being a food snob

I love to drink a flute of sparkling mineral water
    before dinner
I love being as slim as the actresses in French movies
I barely think about food when it's not mealtime
I never feel hungry between meals anymore
I am like someone half my age because I feel so light
    and have abundant energy
I enjoy drinking green tea
Sugary foods make me feel unwell and I much prefer
    to eat three proper meals a day instead
A big glass of water fills me up when I think I'm
    hungry between meals
I am effortlessly slim today and always
Why not me? I can be skinny too – proper Paris
    skinny
I love looking sexy in a bikini at the beach or by the
    pool

I am in *love* with my affirmations. Over time I have added to them, and I feel inspired and re-motivated whenever I read through them. They reset my mind onto the right path when I can feel it wandering off. They remind me why I am doing this. You can find my full list (yes, there are even more!) in the chapter '*Day 28. The magic of slimming affirmations*'.

Steal mine, write ones that are personal to you and build up a reservoir of inspiration for yourself. I saved my affirmations in a Word document and sent them to my Kindle (you can get your Kindle email address from the Kindle settings area on Amazon) so I had them like a book available to read privately anywhere.

Some of the affirmations will be true for you now, and others will be true for the *future you*. Mix them in together to convince your mind that they are all true. When I wrote 'It is okay for me to have three healthy meals a day without snacking', it was *far* from okay. I couldn't imagine getting through one day without eating between meals.

Then one day I did it, and I survived. It was uncomfortable at first and those stretches of time between meals seemed so long, but I distracted myself, sipped water, did jobs, read a book. And then it was my next mealtime.

Making even one affirmation come true for you will give you the confidence that you *can* change and you *can* create truth from your thoughts.

Nourishment = a happy mind

Good food is another way to raise your vibration, in particular protein. Several years ago, I had a few sessions with a personal trainer, and part of his service was evaluating my food. So, I wrote down what I ate for the week and took my sheet of paper nervously along to our next appointment. Glancing at my hand-writing he said 'yep, not enough protein in your meals, most women are like that'.

From that encounter, I now make sure I have a serving of protein with each of my three meals. Having enough protein keeps you full and helps you feel grounded. When I have had meals with no protein in the past I have become jittery and hungry within an hour or two. It's not fun, and certainly does not help with a high frequency.

Eating a chicken and avocado salad for lunch certainly sets me up for a more productive and enjoyable afternoon than if I'd had something junky and low protein like I used to. When I worked at an office in the city I never took my own lunch. Most days I'd buy salmon and avocado sushi, which was fine; but I also 'treated' myself to worse options and then snacked on sweets all afternoon.

On those days, my vibration was at rock-bottom and you can guess I did not go home to cook a healthy vegetable-packed stir-fry; no, it was the fish-and-chip shop which beckoned me when I hopped off the bus.

I have heard of scientific studies which show that the more servings of fruit and vegetables children eat, the happier they feel. I know myself when I am eating healthier I feel better, and when I'm eating badly I feel revolting.

With food you are either on an upward or a downward spiral, depending on what you choose.

In the beginning I had to force myself to choose 'boring' healthy options over the more appealing (at that time) junkier 'treat' options. Now, I love my healthy food and it is rare that I will eat processed foods.

I don't often get headaches now and I feel incredibly vibrant and energetic on a daily basis; happy too. All of this points to a high vibration because *I feel good*, and it is all because of real, healthy fresh fruits and vegetables.

I used to complicate eating so much, but it doesn't need to be complex. In fact, the simpler the better, and it will lead you to amazing places.

Your *Thirty Slim Days* action tips:

Collect together and write your own **mantras, sayings and affirmations**. Keep them in handy places – on an index card in your wallet; have one memorized and repeat it to yourself; gather a whole bunch together and make your own Kindle book to read a little bit of regularly – there are endless possibilities.

Set up **messages on your phone** to be sent at random times if you can do that.

Recording **affirmations in your own voice** and playing them as you exercise or do housework is an excellent way for them to sink in effortlessly too (I keep them private with earphones if my husband is at home).

Remind yourself that **the higher the quality of your food, the better you will feel**. It may not seem that way at first – when I decided to have some time away from sugar, I had the worst headache for four days. I felt tired the whole time and my skin was tender to the touch.

On day five, I woke up like I was in a movie with the sun shining through the window and little birds and mice helping me do my housework, like in the *Enchanted* movie. I felt reborn! From then on, I haven't looked back.

I used to think I enjoyed the 'fun' foods in bags, packets and boxes and I'm sure I did at the time, but I didn't enjoy how I felt. Now I am on the other side I can't see myself going back. The cost is simply too high and I would rather feel **healthy and vibrant** instead. And you can too.

Day 8

Every little action counts

I wanted to write this book about slimming and weight loss for a long time, however I didn't feel qualified. I wanted to have it all figured out *before* I started, but then I realized I might never write this book if that was the case.

I knew I had valuable information and a unique point of view (like we all do). I wanted to share what I already knew and had observed from others, and what worked for me. I also knew deep down that writing this book would help me too.

It made such a difference when I realized I didn't need to be the expert; I could simply add my voice to the conversation around body issues and eating. With that in mind I started writing this book and figured out the rest as I went along.

I do believe that we already have everything inside of us that we need to know, and it's by asking ourselves questions that we can bring out that knowledge. It's also important not to wait until we know everything (when will that be, when we are 97?); because if we try to be perfect, how will we ever learn?

You don't need to be perfect

In this chapter I want to let you know that it's not necessary to be superwoman. You don't have to decide to be a clean eater and perfect about it from here on in. You don't have to *wait* to be perfect before you can consider yourself a success in weight loss or any other part of your life.

All you have to do is make small, incremental changes most days. Aiming for betterment instead of perfection is not only more doable, it's more enjoyable.

You might feel that tiny changes most days is not enough though. That it's not even worth bothering trying because you have too much weight to lose or you've tried before and ended up going back to the way you were.

I get it; I've felt the same more times than I can count. It felt pointless doing ten sit-ups a day and having a small-size latte rather than the large one when my jeans were so tight and I felt like nothing would ever change.

Eating habits change slowly – don't expect miracles

Nothing might change *today*, but over time you will see change. The shape, size, flexibility and strength of your body as it is right now comes as a result of what you have done or not done in the past. But the past is gone and it's not coming back; you can't go back in time and change your habits and daily actions.

What you can do is change what you do today, and every day. Then, in the future your body will reflect all those little betterments you are practising right now. Isn't this a fantastic opportunity we all have? That we can change our body right now, starting today?

We don't even have to look or feel different to know that it's working. All we have to do is follow the process and the outcome will take care of itself. The sorts of small incremental changes I'm talking about are making choices such as:

Moving for fifteen minutes a day – going for a walk, dancing or doing your own fun and silly aerobics moves to three songs in a row, or following a fifteen-minute YouTube workout.

Drinking more water – have a pad of paper on the kitchen counter or maybe there's even an app for your phone, to count off ten glasses a day.

Setting your ideal wake and sleep times – and sticking to them.

Deciding to watch one television program instead of three after dinner – and using the extra time to practice self-care such as giving yourself a facial or organizing your closet.

Not giving up – this is probably the most important, I feel, because if you never give up, you will get there. You only fail when you stop trying; it's not a motivational poster, it's the truth.

Some days you will feel perfect and that's exciting; however there will be other days where you'll feel like it is an uphill battle to get where you thought you wanted to go.

On those days you won't care about your goal weight or your benchmark jeans fitting. You won't care that you want to feel peaceful about your eating. All you will want to do is eat. And eat. And eat.

I had just such a day recently and it was tough going. I was hungry between meals with a hollow feeling inside, despite not being physically hungry. I knew it was addictive food cravings and I didn't want to give in to them because then they would continue to rule me.

I practiced the technique in my chapter '*Day 14. Who are you going to feed?*' and it seemed that all day long I was saying to myself 'Am I going to listen to the addict?' I said it so much I was worried the magic of it would wear off and I'd be left with nothing!

Yes, I really felt that desperate. Even though I had had a good breakfast – scrambled eggs on toast; then I'd had some fruit and a decent handful of raw nuts for a light lunch because I wasn't that hungry after the eggs, I still wanted to eat.

It wasn't healthy food I was craving either. I wanted to go down to the supermarket, buy chocolate, sweets and who knows what else and sit on the sofa scoffing it all, while reading my book.

But I also knew that I *didn't* want that at the same time as wanting it badly. When I've done this in the past I've felt wretched – blobby, ashamed and regretful.

And I also know that I would put myself right back at square one in terms of dealing with those cravings; because if you feed them they will remain strong. If you can manage *not* to feed them; over time they will go away and you won't have to deal with them ever again.

So for three or four hours I was literally hanging on by the skin of my teeth; making it to dinnertime when I could eat my dinner, drink a cup of tea and go to bed, because tomorrow is always a new start.

I ended up having a small nap later in the day, before dinner. In the past when I've given in to the cravings I wished I would have done this; instead of eating something to give me energy I could have listened to my body and rested.

Overall I did not eat perfectly that day – I had a small amount of cheese and crackers after my light lunch, then a little while after that I had a medium-sized bowl of potato chips and a can of soft drink while I read a book.

In the past I would have been angry at myself that I'd 'given in', but comparing that to how I could have eaten, I definitely feel like I did well.

My old defeatist thinking would have kicked in in the past as well. If I had considered that day a failure, I would have told myself, *I knew I couldn't stick with it, I may as well not bother because I am always going to be the same. I may as well face it now.*

My new way of thinking is that I did as well as I could on that day, and I'll do even better next time. Not only is this a more loving way to talk to myself, but it has a better outcome too; there was no rebellion or remorsefulness.

There certainly are days when I could eat a horse for no apparent reason; I don't know why, but we are humans, not machines, so lots of different factors will come into play. The weather, hormones, how well we slept – so many that we might not be aware of them all.

What I do know is that on those days the best you can do is minimise the damage. And, be thankful for small wins, like I was. **Take small imperfect actions every day**. Some days will be more imperfect than others, and that's okay.

Your *Thirty Slim Days* action tips:

Be forgiving of yourself when you perceive a day to have been less than perfect.

Aim for small upgrades and betterments each day, instead of quantum leaps.

Keep on going. You might think that the changes you are making are too small to make a difference, but they're not. Everything you do that is heading in the direction counts, no matter how small that step is.

Know that it doesn't matter how far down the wrong road you've come, **you can turn around at any time.**

Day 9

Address your danger times

It is not necessary to overhaul your entire life and turn everything upside down in order to lose weight and become healthier. It's a tempting thing to do and very alluring, because we all love the complete makeover and big reveal of something like this.

But how has this approach worked for you in the past? I know for me, it hasn't, because I've invariably gone back to the way I was before, and put the weight back on, plus a little more for good measure. Over time, my upper level of weight has increased and now, looking back ten or fifteen years; what was once my 'fat' weight I would be happy to be that weight now.

I know there is scientific proof that your metabolism slows down over the years; hormonal shifts making it harder to lose weight around the middle among other similarly depressing statistics.

For me, I choose not to believe these kinds of statements, because they don't feel good and I don't want to use them as excuses either. Of course, we can't change our hormones, our age or our gender. What I choose to focus on though, is what I *can* change.

Did you know there is other scientific proof that what we believe to be factual ends up coming true for us? That we can actually make ourselves feel healthier or sicker by what we believe to be true? You must have heard of the placebo effect. Who knows what is really the correct answer, so why don't we believe all the good stuff and go from there. If nothing else, it just feels a lot better.

When I am working with what I can change and what I do have control over, I find it helpful to look through my day or my week, and see where the times are that I go out-of-control.

You may wish to keep a journal to identify the problem areas, but I already know when mine are – late afternoon and weekends. These are the times I feel like I've earned the right to kick back and relax with a book or magazine and some treats to nibble on.

The issue is, I don't stop at a small portion. I am enjoying myself so much that I continue on and end up stuffing myself.

Why do we eat at certain times?

I have asked myself, *Why? Why can't I stop at one portion and then leave a nice, long gap until my meal is ready? Why do I snack continuously, sometimes right up until food is on my plate at dinnertime?*

The answer is that I love the time-out; I love treating myself; I love that I can do that if I want to – there are no parents to tell me I am going to spoil my dinner. It's a habit that I look forward to... but I also hate it at the same time.

As humans, we are biologically programmed to seek pleasure and avoid pain. It is instinctual. I obviously connect more pleasure to the eating of my favourite treat foods than I do to the pain of being too full to enjoy my dinner and also the pain of not fitting my clothes well.

My favoured down-time links together our lovely comfy sofas, a book or magazine and some yummy snacks. I tried to combine the sofa and book or magazine without snacks, but it was torture. I didn't even last a minute! I have these links so firmly entrenched in my mind and every time I do it, I am strengthening that connection.

I tried giving myself little jobs from 4-6pm such as doing a load of laundry, addressing a small decluttering task or working on a sewing or knitting project, but I don't really have the energy later in the day. I'd rather do jobs in the morning or early afternoon.

I wanted to break the link between sofa-reading-snacking while still enjoying some down-time, and came up with an excellent solution that rolled two desires into one.

Change your surroundings to change your habits

My boudoir time which used to be after dinner for an hour or so, had gradually disappeared. There wasn't really a reason; I let my after-dinner time linger on, then it was time to get ready for bed.

Ideally I wanted to fit in an hour between dinner clean-up and bedtime to journal, read *Victoria* magazine or my current fiction book, and maybe apply a facemask while sipping herbal tea. I wanted to do this a few times each week but it had ended up not even being a few times a month.

In addition, I wanted to create a relaxing late-afternoon ritual. So, I combined the two and decided to have pre-dinner boudoir time. I have never eaten in my bedroom, so it is not linked to food. I could read or journal relaxing on our bed with a drink – I like a flute of sparkling lemon or lime Perrier – and in doing so, disrupt my pre-dinner snacking habit.

I am happy to report the change of venue has been a cracking success, and I have also found a second place to relax with my book which does not trigger my nibbles either. In the summer it is quite warm in our upstairs bedroom. Stepping out our back door off the laundry one day, I noticed how cool and breezy it was on the tiny balcony.

This side of the house gets sun in the morning and then is shaded from mid-afternoon onwards. It was the perfect place to take my drink and book outside and enjoy the cool breeze at the hottest time of the day. I take a cushion to sit on and have even had the cats join me most days.

Over time it has become the norm for me not to eat before dinner; just like I have done before with a morning coffee and muffin habit on the way to work at my office job in the city. I would walk past my favourite coffee place and pick up one of their delicious apricot and almond muffins and a café latte to enjoy when I arrived at the office. It turned from an occasional treat into something I craved every day at one stage.

I eventually left that job to work with my husband in our retail footwear business, and didn't miss that morning muffin; it was simply part of my routine in that job.

Your routines are what make or break you – they can strengthen or weaken you

With my late afternoon sofa routine, I have changed my location which naturally leads me away from nibbling since I never eat in our bedroom. A cup of tea in the morning, herbal tea at night or a flute of sparkling water during my new, earlier boudoir time, yes. Food, no.

If I'd had this thought during my muffin-morning-time, I may have started a new morning routine such as going for a half-hour stroll before work or even taking a different route to the office, which did not involve going past that café with its delicious muffins.

When I think about it now, it's so simple, but sometimes it's hard to see a message that is so clearly staring you in the face.

Look at your danger times – when are they?

If you need to, go ahead and start a log where you track your eating for at least a week, preferably three. Or, simply step back through the previous month and see if there were times that you know you were not in complete control.

Maybe it is after a regular appointment where your favourite food outlet is close by, and your standing appointment is at lunchtime. Can you change the location or the time of your appointment? The food that tempts you at noon might not look so appealing if your new appointment time is 9am.

I used to meet a friend for Saturday afternoon movies for a while, and it was hard for me to resist the popcorn. We both joined Weight Watchers at the same time and I remember one day we brought along a small bag each of crumbled rice cakes as a lower calorie substitute. What a depressing outing that was!

Then I had the idea for us to go to a more stylish cinema, which served espresso coffee rather than having a big popcorn machine belching out yellow-coated kernels. Because of the rarefied atmosphere and pleasant lingering aroma of coffee, I didn't even miss the popcorn and had no desire to bring my own baggie of crumbs.

Instead I was the elegant and dignified woman of my dreams, sipping on my coffee or small bottle of sparkling mineral water. It was a much better feeling. Switching up our previous blockbuster-type movie place with loud noises and that revolting yet strangely alluring popcorn smell to a more civilized theatre where even the clientele were of a higher class, was a fantastic switch. The type of movies were far superior also.

Happily, I have not bought popcorn or any snacks at the movies for a number of years now, and I don't feel like I am missing out. When I saw the James Bond movie *Spectre* with my husband last year, we planned to go out for dinner afterwards. In the past that would not stop me from having popcorn, but because I had trained myself out of the popcorn habit, I wasn't tempted at all.

Change can happen effortlessly

This proves to me that habits and behaviours that you think are *fixed* and *forever*, are not. You need to give yourself a chance to forget about them by changing some part of your routine or ritual.

The human brain loves to feel comfortable, and repeating old habits is relaxing because your brain knows what to expect. That's why it can be hard to change a habit – you feel discomfort so your brain says, *Let's go back to the way things were,* even if the old habit was making you unhappy.

If you choose small adjustments, change will be easier and longer-lasting. This is because your slight changes feel comfortable to your mind – less disruptive.

Hypnotherapist Marisa Peer says to **make the familiar unfamiliar, and the unfamiliar familiar**. You aren't stuck in your own habits and helpless under your cravings and danger times. You just need to change what is familiar in your life.

Your *Thirty Slim Days* action tips:

Have a session **brainstorming possible swaps** for your danger times. Write everything down that you can think of and don't talk yourself out of recording them. I have found my best ideas in the silliest notes I've written for myself; and sometimes you need to let them marinate a little bit to receive what you need to from them.

Habits and triggers can be the time of day as with my pre-dinner danger time; they can be situational, as with my movie popcorn; and they can be people-related (you always overeat with a certain friend).

Ask yourself:

What your danger times are?

Why you think you overeat or eat junk at these times; what do you gain from your behaviour?

Possible changes you could make, so that you don't indulge in the behaviour you are trying to eliminate.

Find out a way to turn around your thinking so that you actively choose the new option instead of feeling like it is being forced on you (the simple act of saying 'I choose this...' is powerful).

Choose to feel good about your change.

Practice your change over and over; if you find yourself tempted to fall back into old habits, say to yourself 'that was the old me, the new me does it this way...'

It was quite exciting to me when I saw that by changing one or two danger times, I was vastly improving my daily experience. Not everything in my life was broken; all I needed were a few minor adjustments.

Day 10
Le regime chic

This book is mostly about the mindset of a slim person, however I wanted to write a chapter about how I eat, because I'm sure some of you will be curious. I certainly am when it comes to ladies I know or have seen in the media; I'm always keen to see exactly what and how they eat.

Sometimes it is simple nosiness, but often I think they might know a magical secret I've never heard of. From what I have seen, the magical secret to being slim and healthy is to have chic portion sizes and eat mostly healthy food, with very little processed food.

But that would make an unacceptably short chapter, wouldn't it?

In this chapter I will go through what I eat on a regular day, and how I arrived at that. Of course, my menus will change over time, but for the most part the basics are the same.

I have tried my fair share of diets in the past. What has worked best for me is to create my own eating plan using inspiration and ideas I gather along the way.

A couple of months before I turned forty (I am forty-six as I write this book), I came up with a set of food guidelines which I christened *Le Regime Chic*. In 2010, when I first wrote them, I had been sharing my food journey on my blog *How to be Chic* as I attempted to lose weight.

But I sometimes had off-weeks where I hadn't been 'good', and there wasn't anything particularly noteworthy to report.

To take the pressure off, I relaxed and thought to myself, 'How can I change this? How can I get back onto a good track with regards to food, eating and my weight?' It was still 'No' to Weight Watchers (too strict for me and I would rebel); but giving myself free rein was a recipe for disaster.

I drew up guidelines for the way I wanted to live; guidelines to enable me to slim down slowly and quietly. They were not a diet, and no quantities were listed. I simply daydreamed how my week would look in a perfect and relaxed world.

Here are my original guidelines (at the time I called them 'Countdown to 40', just for fun):

Sunday to Thursday – alcohol-free nights

*Friday night – Bubbly Friday (we've had Bubbly
    Friday for years)*
Saturday night – snacks and drinks

*This means I've cut down drinks to two nights a week
    (from probably 5-7 nights, even one glass of wine
    each evening adds up to a lot of calories) and I
    only eat snacks one night a week. I've decided I
    would rather have some camembert and crackers
    than potato chips, but if I want potato chips that's
    fine too, but only on Saturdays.*

Salad with lunch every day
Vegetables with dinner every night

Protein at every meal, e.g.:
- Egg with breakfast
- Tuna with lunch
- Lean meat or fresh fish with dinner

One piece of fresh fruit every day

*If I crave something sweet after a meal – 1-2 squares
    dark chocolate*
*If I crave savoury snacks, a small amount of rice
    crackers and cheese*

*Early nights – in bed by 9.30pm at the latest,
    preferably 9pm, to give plenty of boudoir time for*

reading and moisturizing before lights out at 10pm.

Green tea first thing in the morning with blog time (6am)
Drink water all day

Two yoga classes per week
Three one-hour walks per week

Having these guidelines helped me to stay on track and enjoy a balanced lifestyle, with plenty of nutrition and good sleep.

I liked that they were not only about food, but incorporated lifestyle habits I wanted to aim for as well. I also used my original Chic Eating principles most of the time (I can have anything I like as long as it is 'Chic' and 'Real').

If I ever felt like slacking off, maybe pouring a glass of wine on a Wednesday, I remembered my *Countdown to 40* list and felt newly remotivated. I also had the Word document open on my laptop most of the time, so I could see it whenever I was on the computer.

Last year I revisited and updated *Le Regime Chic*. It has changed a bit, because I no longer drink alcohol. I stopped almost five years ago; I've written about this on my blog if you are interested in reading about it – go to howtobechic.com and type non-drinker into the search box on the top-left of the screen.

Plus I was diagnosed as celiac a few years back so I am now completely wheat- and gluten-free, doctor's orders! Taking these factors into account, my current version of *Le Regime Chic* is as follows:

Monday to Friday – snack-free nights – enjoy Perrier in a champagne flute
Saturday and Sunday nights – snacks and drinks – Copper Kettle potato chips, only buy one bag per week, with my chosen drinks.

Fruit for breakfast most days (sometimes eggs)
Salad with lunch every day
Vegetables with dinner every night

Protein at every meal, e.g.:
- Raw nuts with breakfast
- Cold roast meat, eggs or canned fish with lunch
- Lean meat or fresh fish with dinner

Avocado every day, half or one, usually with lunch

If I crave something sweet after a meal – 1-2 squares dark chocolate
If I crave savoury snacks, handful of dry-roasted unsalted nuts

Early nights – computer off by dinner time, in bed by 9.30pm at the latest, preferably 9pm, to give plenty of boudoir time for reading and moisturizing before lights out at 10pm.

Drink water all day – tick off ten glasses before 6pm

Think 'What can I eat for maximum nutrition?'

Hot black tea with trim milk first thing in the morning with writing time (6am)
Drink water all day

One or two weight-bearing workouts at home or yoga classes per week
Three forty-five minute walks per week
(these are alternated, so I am doing something active five or six days a week)

An example of a day's *Le Regime Chic* meal for me is:

Breakfast – either chopped fresh fruit, a handful or raw nuts and a soy café latte, or poached/soft-boiled eggs (two or three) on a piece of gluten-free toast (sometimes with butter, sometimes not) and a soy café latte

Mid-morning – a cup of tea

Lunch – a big salad with protein such as cold roast chicken or other roast meat, two or three hard-boiled eggs (not if I had eggs for breakfast though) or a can of tuna or salmon.

In the winter I might have left-over chicken curry or spaghetti bolognaise (without the pasta). I like to make soup, but I also need protein at lunchtime and many of my favourite soups are vegetarian such as pumpkin or tomato soup, so I make a side salad with protein to have with them. Occasionally I might have a small portion of cheese and crackers alongside my soup instead.

After lunch – a bliss ball and a coffee with creamy milk

Mid-late afternoon – a champagne flute of sparkling mineral water (I love lemon or lime Perrier) or a sugar-free Red Bull (not too often though)

I do still have potato chips as a treat, so I try not to have them every day - it's easier when I follow my chapter *'Day 14. Who are you going to feed?'* I have one small dish and the remainder of the bag put away sealed before I sit down. I also sometimes buy the kiddie packets and have one of those, although saying that makes think 'what am I eating kiddie food for...' Something to address another day!

Dinner – usually a protein such as chicken or steak, maybe fish, with lots of fresh green vegetables, and not too many starchy vegetables. We cook roasts or mini-roasts in the oven a lot; I also make pasta meals a few times a month and we have steak on the barbeque in the summer.

Often, we will cut back on carbohydrates – potatoes, pasta, rice etc. – while keeping the protein and good fats up (such as avocado on our lunchtime salad) and plenty of green and bright vegetables.

After dinner – I have a coffee with creamy milk and a piece or two of dark chocolate (Lindt 90% cacao is my current favourite); I sometimes have one piece of dark chocolate paired with a bliss ball which tastes quite decadent.

This is a very typical day's eating for me, and I found the hardest thing was not snacking between meals. But if I carried on snacking, particularly in my biggest danger-time of mid-to-late afternoon, nothing would ever change.

I wouldn't take off the weight that made me look and feel frumpy, in fact my weight would likely climb higher over time like it had been. Plus, I would entrench the habit even further.

It was often not easy for me to get through that time of day without succumbing to a snack, but I knew that the more I beat it, the easier it would get. It's not like I was hungry; often I had had lunch with adequate protein only an hour or two before.

No, it was all in my mind and what I had let myself get away with for too long.

Update: *Le Regime Chic* is constantly evolving for me. Even since I wrote these updates a few months ago, I no longer have potato chips which I am very happy about. I found it hard to give them up, but now I think differently about them and I don't have them at all. I simply decided I am not a person who eats them. In addition, they are not chic nor are they real as per my chic eating guidelines!

Having my own *Le Regime Chic* to look to for guidance removed any doubt from my mind. Because I had written it out at a time when I was relaxed and happy, I made good choices.

When you are feeling on the edge about eating something you know will not be beneficial to you, you likely won't make good choices. It is much like writing out a grocery list and sticking to it when you get to the supermarket regardless of what your eyes and stomach tell you.

If you say to yourself 'I'm only buying what's on my list', you won't get there and think 'Ooh, potato chips are on special, maybe I should get a few bags'. Well, Fiona, are they on your shopping list? I didn't think so.

Another way I like to update *Le Regime Chic* with new ideas from time to time, is by brainstorming all the ways I can bring health into my life every day, such as:

Daily Goodness

Walk
Stretch
Journal
10-12 glasses of water
Sleep
I weigh 61kg
Fruit
Vegetables
Protein – eggs, meat, fish, raw nuts
Good fats – avocado
I love being skinny
1 song of aerobics workout
Military/hotel room workout

And sometimes I like to plan a day ahead of time with exact foods I am going to eat, as I did with this journal entry written out the night before. Here's what I planned for and then ate that day:

'Le Regime Chic for tomorrow'

I weigh 61kg

6am – hot English Breakfast tea with trim milk and writing (yes, doing it now!)

I do my at-home-weight bearing workout – 15 minutes, then a shower

Breakfast after my workout: Fresh blueberries, strawberries, peach, nectarine (a medium sized bowl) with a small handful of raw mixed nuts and a small soy latte

Morning tea – a hot cup of Earl Grey tea with trim milk

Lunch – homemade chicken salad, coffee and a bliss ball

Afternoon tea – cheese and crackers (four crackers and four thin slices of cheese), Perrier

Dinner – chicken stir-fried with onion, carrot, broccoli and mushrooms on a small amount of rice with Indonesian curry (gourmet ready-sachet), coffee and Lindt 90% chocolate (one big square)

Stretches

Bedtime at 9pm

I find it so helpful to have a little plan in mind and it makes a big difference the next day. I don't do this all the time; mostly I run on auto-pilot but every so often I like to step through my day the night before.

And lastly, in the journal entry below, I captured a day's eating at the end of the day. I'd had a day where I felt relaxed; I was not obsessing about food; I ate in what felt like a healthy and normal way and I hadn't had any weird cravings or hunger. A total win! So, I wanted to note down what I'd had for future reference, and also record the proof for myself that I could eat in a calm, easy-going and healthful way.

My day:

Hot tea with trim milk first thing

Breakfast - two poached eggs on toast with butter, soy milk café latte

Water, water, water

Lunch - homemade savoury mince with a side salad of celery, carrot and avocado
Vanilla cupcake, coffee

Water, water, water

Lemon Perrier in a flute, small bowl of potato chips

Dinner - roast chicken with loads of vegetables

Two squares of dark chocolate
Decaf coffee

Writing out your own little lists and plans is far preferable to following a meal plan from a magazine or diet company. I think you can take inspiration from these sources and from what others do, but ultimately you will want to create a food and lifestyle plan especially for you.

When you make it **enticing and fun**, you can't wait to get started. Jotting down a whole lot of inspirational notes makes it something to look forward to instead of a diet plan to dread starting on Monday.

Your *Thirty Slim Days* action tips:

Start your own *Le Regime Chic* file, whether it's on a computer document or pen and paper.

Name your outline in a way that makes you feel excited to follow it: choose something elegant. The name *Le Regime Chic* really calls to me. It says 'here is your pathway to being the stylish and slender woman of your dreams'. You are welcome to use this name for your notes, or you might wish to name them something completely different.

If I was to choose a different name, I might go with:

Fiona's Slender and Elegant Life
La Cuisine Chic-Notes
The New Me
Fiona 2.0

Whatever you choose, make sure you find it **fun, appealing, and stylish**. Then you will enjoy creating and following it.

Imagine how a pleasing day's menu would go for you and write this down.

Note all the **self-care items** you'd love to include in an ideal week and how often you would like to do them – daily, weekly, monthly?

Add to your *Le Regime Chic* plan as you think of other habits you want to include, and when you **come across good ideas from others**.

Use your plan as inspiration to bring your **chic daily habits into reality**.

Adjust as you need to and look at what you do and don't do. If there are items on your list that the ideal you does but you still aren't doing, ask yourself why. Perhaps you don't really want to but think you should.

Or maybe you are putting too much pressure on yourself to be perfect. **Perfection isn't necessary** for success, but loving yourself is. Go easy on yourself and repeat the mantra *I am enough, I am doing enough*, when you feel like you aren't getting there.

You are, and it will come.

Day 11

Change one thing at a time

It is always tempting to go for the big makeover and give yourself a life overhaul, all at once. I know because I've done it many times; in fact I even have a Word document entitled 'Lifestyle Overhaul' where I outlined exactly what I was going to do to whip myself into shape.

Yes, that document has virtual cobwebs all over it.

I've found from experience that a far better approach is to choose one thing to change and stick with it... no matter what. You can then choose other habits to change later, maybe in a month, maybe longer; but to start with, have one change to focus on.

Go after what you want with a laser focus

There's an analogy I love about the magnifying glass. If you move around holding a magnifying glass, it is harmless. But if you hold it in one place long enough with the sun streaming through it, you can set a piece of paper alight. This shows that if you focus on one thing with a laser-like intensity, you are almost guaranteed to achieve it.

Remembering this analogy always gives me good motivation to *focus* and *persevere*. You really can accomplish anything if you keep it top of mind for long enough.

Think back to school when you had an assignment due – if you left it until the last minute you had no choice but to work on that assignment to the exclusion of all else. And did you get it finished? Of course you did.

Laser focus equally applies to what you want... and what you don't want. If your focus is on how heavy you feel and all the foods you can't eat and still be skinny, you will sooner or later indulge in those foods. Before too long you will be back to the way you were.

If, however, you focus on all the delicious healthy foods you now nourish your body with, how good you are going to feel being thinner and how much you are looking forward to fitting your favourite smaller-size clothes; you are much more likely to stay the distance.

Focusing on what you don't want brings about feelings of misery and deprivation. Focusing on the desired outcome brings you feelings of excitement and anticipation. Which do you think sounds more enticing?

Find your anchor habit

Over time I have changed many habits for the better using this method. In addition, I also have one anchor habit that I go back to when I find myself slipping into unhelpful ways. My anchor habit is 'no sugar'. This is the habit that when I break it, everything else goes out the window. Sugar is my biggest vice.

My version of 'no sugar' is 'hardly any sugar'. There are some sweet food items that I can happily eat in moderation and I include those in my diet. I can easily have a shop-bought cake in the pantry and have a slender slice after lunch or dinner. I can take or leave it and have days in between with no cake.

Home baking is not so easy to resist, so I tend not to bake much. Once I was diagnosed as celiac I threw away my (small) baking stash because it was unsafe for me, and I have not gone out of my way to replace it with the gluten-free versions.

When we have guests, I love to make a fruit crumble for dessert, so I have bought ingredients for that; and I make bliss balls so I have dried dates and apricots, but that's about it.

'No sugar' means I don't buy lollies/sweets/candy, cheap milk chocolate, ice-cream and other juvenile food like that. When I do, I go off the rails with my eating, so keeping that one rule in mind is helpful to me.

It might be something else for you – perhaps bread, potatoes or savoury junk food.

Say your worst vice is the golden arches but you don't really care so much for other brands of fast food. Your anchor habit that you keep in place or come back to if you stray could be 'no McDs'.

You can have any of the other brands if you really want it; sometimes you will and sometimes you won't. Doing this means you don't feel so deprived because you aren't saying no to everything at once.

This is exactly what my brother did when I met up with him at a food court recently When I asked if he was having his favourite McDonalds for lunch, he replied, 'Nope, I don't eat that anymore'. He still ate at the food court, he just chose something different rather than forcing himself to sit at home with a cold salad as the alternative. I was seriously impressed with the meal he chose too, stacked high with healthy vegetables.

This is also how I run my 'no sugar' rule. If I want some potato chips, I can have them. If I want to buy some gluten-free biscuits/cookies to have, that's fine. I know that with both of those foods I can have one small serving and be happy with it.

You will know what foods you can keep and what foods you will be better off kicking out of your life. Just ask yourself what foods you cannot stop at just one bite.

What are the goodies that you must finish the bag or container and you could still go back for more? List them all down and pick your worst one to have as your anchor habit. When your anchor habit has been successful for a while – at least a month – you can introduce another habit that you'd like to change.

If you find that you've been thrown off and have returned to your worst vice, go back to focusing on your anchor habit. It doesn't mean you are a failure if you do this repeatedly; it means you are *human*.

I have had times when I've felt like an utter failure because I landed back at square one, even while writing this book; but who said I was a failure? Only me. Remembering one of my favourite motivational quotes helps me continue: *You are only a failure if you quit. If you keep going despite stumbling, you are not a failure.*

Choose your ideal lifestyle habits

Many habits I'd like to change aren't necessarily directly related to health and slimness, but are related to wellness and happiness as well. To me these are all interlinked.

Brainstorm a big list and include everything you can think of that would make your life happier, easier, slimmer and healthier. Choose the one that you think would make the most difference overall and make that your anchor habit. Highlight it or put it at the top of your page.

Some of mine are:

No sugar
Three meals, no snacking
Drink more water
Lights out at 10pm, rise at 6am
Walk daily
Resistance training three times each week
Plan out meals in advance
Grocery shop for the week
Get showered/dressed/hair/bit of makeup even if I'm at home for the day
Don't buy any groceries that my ideal self would not purchase – if it's not in my home it's harder for me to eat it
Clean and organize my pantry once a week
Keep my grooming habits up
Journal daily
Nothing accumulates on the dining table, it is cleared at least once daily
Create a list of home projects that I want to complete – decluttering, fixing up, tidying, reorganizing, sorting areas that bother me

Some habits are smaller and can be slipped into your daily schedule easily, while others will need to be a focused effort to have them become second-nature.

For me, water is something that I love to drink, but sometimes I notice I have not had as much as I usually do. If this is the case I make sure to always have a big glass on the desk beside me or keep a glass by the tap in the kitchen so I have a drink of water every time I am pass by.

That's an easy habit for me to re-instigate without rocking the boat too much. Likewise grooming. I have upgraded my grooming habits so that I now moisturize my entire body every single day. I never miss a day; it's as engrained as brushing my teeth.

Flossing is another habit I have been successful with too. Years ago my dentist asked if I flossed. I used to hate that question because I didn't floss at all when I was younger. I answered 'yes', and he asked 'how often?' When I said 'probably 29 out of 30 days but usually 30/30' he was shocked. 'That's more than I do', he said.

Certain parts of my grooming I have practiced until they are second nature, but I have some such as blow-drying my hair nicely or shaving my legs that I put off if I can get away with it. I decided to give myself a break by getting my legs waxed, and I have been much better blow-drying my hair. I thought this was a good compromise.

I notice that when I let those parts of my grooming slip, other seemingly unrelated areas in my life slacken as well. So, by keeping up those little, easy habits I feel like other self-improvements are more achievable.

What could those daily habits do for you in a year?

Imagine if in twelve months' time you had layered all the small habits on your list. After a year would you be the same person you are now, or do you think you might have changed? Another way to look at this, is to ask yourself 'If I looked back a year from now and had changed only one thing, what would make the most difference to my life?'

Even if you change one habit only and don't add any others, you would notice a huge difference in a year. I know for me that 'no sugar' reaps health, happiness and financial benefits even if I do not change anything else.

Your *Thirty Slim Days* action tips:

Make a list of every positive habit you think would make a difference to your daily life. Firstly choose your anchor habit. If you can't see one easily, that's okay; leave it for later. Like cream in milk, it will float to the top. At some stage you will realize there is that one habit that when you let it slip away, everything else goes to pieces.

Choose one habit to maintain, and layer other habits over top of it. You can do an intensive course choosing one habit a day for a month. My friend Stephanie did this with great results. Or if that feels too fast (I couldn't sustain daily for long, less than two weeks), try one a week or one a month.

Print out a calendar page (I use the calendar in Excel) and write your new habit along the top. Cross off each day as you are successful. Apparently Jerry Seinfeld did this with his career.

When asked how he had managed to come up with episode after episode of high quality television with his series *Seinfeld*, he replied that he wrote a joke every day. Once he had finished his new material for that day, he crossed the day off on his calendar. He loved seeing rows of crossed days and didn't want to see a gap, so he kept on going.

Day 12
Become someone who does not snack

I have heard the famous 'how to be a French girl' advice of *no snacking* so often that it almost washes over me without effect now. Every list of *10 ways to eat like a Parisian* includes this snippet. I tried it once or twice but it was hard and I don't think I lasted even a day. I thought I was going to die if I didn't have a snack to tide me over when it was still two hours until dinner-time.

Sometimes I would have a healthy snack of apple slices and raw almonds as a snack, but more often it would be a large packet of kettle chips. If I was trying to be healthier I would portion control my kettle chips.

But not snack, ever? I couldn't handle it. It wasn't even a matter of waiting until I was hungry. Occasionally I wanted to eat something straight after a meal, for goodness sake. So to try and tell me not to eat for five or more hours in a row? Well, don't even go there.

I know there are people with medical conditions which requires them to eat every few hours. I am not one of them. I am in perfect health according to the annual blood test report I receive each year (well, almost perfect except for low iron from my celiac status).

I specifically asked the doctor about my blood sugar results one time, convinced that there was a reason for my needing to snack. Nope, it turned out my blood sugar was fine. There really was no other reason for my between-meal snacking than:

It is a habit because I have done it for so long
I am a piglet sometimes
I love to eat
I don't like saying no to myself
I like to taste yummy food

Our friend, leptin

There is also the issue of leptin. Leptin is a hormone we all have in our body which burns fat and also tells us when we are full. One way that this hormone can be blocked is by snacking between meals. When leptin is blocked, we do not burn fat; we also do not have a cut-off switch while eating.

For leptin to work well, we must allow five to six hours, but at least a bare minimum of four, to elapse between meals. You can't do this when snacking, even in a healthy way.

By eating three meals a day with no snacks in between, you will eventually find a cut-off point where you don't want to eat any more. I used to wonder why I didn't have a cut-off point and I thought that some people did and some didn't.

This is a very simplistic explanation; there is more to leptin than that. When I first read about leptin I was horrified that health professionals say to have healthy snacks between meals when it is not beneficial to our bodies.

And of course the food types make a difference too. I didn't have a cut-off point for chocolate, but I did for salad. It wasn't like I finished a big lunch salad and then said 'oh I could keep on eating this all day', but I would think that with chocolate.

And burning fat while you sleep? Just another side effect of having healthy leptin levels. Well, who wouldn't want that.

I did it, and... I survived

So, one day I decided to try it. I decided to become one of those unicorn non-snacking people. It would require planning, preparation and perseverance. I knew after the initial phase that it would become routine for me, and I was looking forward to it that.

I made sure my meals were big enough, because that's something I would need to address. Prior to this decision I would have the tiniest portion convincing myself it was chic to do so, or else not have enough protein (or any, sometimes). Protein is vital at mealtimes because it keeps you satisfied for longer (and it also prevent sugar cravings – yay!)

I planned my filling and healthy meals with plenty of fresh fruit and vegetables, a small amount of fat and a normal portion of protein (a palm-size piece of chicken or steak; or two eggs for example). I enjoyed my meal then... got on with my day.

It wasn't as easy as all that though. I had many uncomfortable moments when I desperately wanted to eat something but knew that I would have to wait until my next meal.

When I was asked myself whether I was hungry in my stomach the answer was always no; except for maybe an hour prior to my next meal, in which case I had a glass of water and busied myself while I waited for that meal.

I wasn't hungry but I Just. Wanted. To. Eat. Something. It sounds so ludicrous to say it, but I liked chewing. I wanted something fun to taste. I wanted to relax and I definitely didn't feel relaxed. Chocolate-covered almonds would relax me! But no, they were not a meal component and I no longer snacked.

It's quite incredible how much I learned in those first weeks of not snacking.

Here are some of my lessons:

I was never in danger of dying
I was thirsty half the time so a glass of water fixed that
I talked myself down from the ledge successfully... a
  lot
I was fully capable of eating only three meals a day
  with nothing else
The discomfort was more mental than physical
I took a few naps in the late afternoon

This last one was quite fascinating to me. Between 4pm and 6pm was my worst snacking time.

Take note of your natural daily cycles

In an article on circadian rhythms, 3.30pm is pinpointed timewise as a dip in energy, coming back up at 6pm and dipping back down after dinner. This is the time I would most often snack, even if I hadn't snacked anywhere else in the day; and that was the time I found the hardest to get through when I stopped snacking.

I wonder if this is why I craved something to snack on at this time of the day? To give myself more energy? When I was dipping into a bag of something yummy (and unhealthy), I would sometimes think *Wouldn't it be better if I simply rested at this time, rather than try and give myself energy with junk food?*

Well of course I never listened to that voice; it was far more fun to eat whatever I wanted, and those foods *taste good* because they are designed to tempt our tastebuds so we'll want more.

When my favourite snack foods were no longer an option in the afternoon, I was forced to look around for other solutions. I didn't write much at this time because I couldn't even think straight. So, once all my jobs were done – the washing was folded, dishwasher emptied and our house tidied, I'd sit down with a book to read and a glass of Perrier.

It was a bit grim to start with, but I'm okay now because I am more used to it. But I found myself getting sleepy sometimes, especially in the beginning – I could barely keep my eyes open. Instead of fighting it (no chance) or eating to prop myself up artificially, I did what seemed most natural.

Even though I felt like the laziest person in the world the few times I did it, I put my bookmark in and closed my eyes. Sometimes on the sofa, sometimes on our bed. I would wake up an hour or so later and magically it was dinner-time.

I knew I had been spoiling myself for too long by snacking whenever I wanted and it was to my detriment. I had frumpy-looking extra weight hanging around and I knew all the processed foods weren't making my body happy.

Work *with* your body – she keeps asking you to!

Imagine your poor body having to work out what to do with all those plastic-looking foods when it has evolved to process real food. At its simplest, our body is a sophisticated machine designed to run on natural food-stuffs. It takes in a piece of fruit, for example; extracts all the nutrients, fibre and water; then gets rid of what it can't utilize.

What do you think it says when you feed it a cheese-flavoured yellow whatever? *Help! That's not in the manual!* probably.

Our bodies are actually very clever, and they can get around our terrible diets. They will work hard to extract what nutrients there are from almost anything. But, and here's the horrible part: there are no nutrients in processed foods.

Processed foods are like the pieces of plastic that sea turtles and marine life eat thinking they are food; trash which fills up their stomach and they think they are full. But they become malnourished and ill, because they have had nothing their body can use for energy and good health.

I know that's not a very nice story, I used to hate seeing those pictures when I watched the news; but it's what we are doing to our bodies by snacking on processed foods. And once I stopped snacking, my processed food consumption plummeted. Snack foods are rarely part of a meal.

It's crazy that companies have become highly profitable from building up a category of food that should not even exist. There are novelty chocolate bars marketed as helping you through a snack attack, and snack-size portions of potato chips available.

Not-snacking magically cures a lot of other things

Deciding not to snack, and to eat only three times a day – which actually is plenty when you think about it. Three times! Every single day! – meant I didn't have to say 'I am never eating salted peanuts, popcorn, candy and cheap chocolate again'.

It naturally started happening because there was no meal I would ever have occasion to eat those things as a component or a side dish. There just wasn't!

I've mentioned already that it wasn't easy in the beginning. Yes, it's true. It was difficult. But I was determined to succeed. Other people do it, so why not me? And as with my other changes, I felt *empowered* not *deprived* by my choice.

When I saw someone else chowing down, I didn't feel envious. I was not depriving myself, I was empowering myself. Snacking held no appeal to me anymore, and it all started with a decision to change.

Now that I have done it for a while, I find it easier and easier to do. It feels normal for me now, whereas when I started it felt normal to graze. I changed what was normal, and you can too.

Your *Thirty Slim Days* action tips:

Do you snack at all, or do you stick to three meals a day? How would you feel if I asked you to consider it? Horrified? Nonplussed? Imagine if you **made this one change and didn't follow any diet or rules**. You couldn't help but be slimmer.

It would mean you would want to **put extra thought into your meals** because you would have to last until your next meal. Moving away from constant snacking – even healthy snacking – might feel hard, but it's worth persevering with.

To paraphrase Og Mandino, *I will persist and I will succeed.*

And so can you.

Day 13
Let your life be easier

One big thing I see over and over, both in myself and other women, is that we do *a lot* at different stages throughout our lives. We might work, look after children, have family obligations, belong to clubs and groups, and generally live amongst constant busy-ness.

School children have after school activities, sports and extra lessons; mothers are driving them around to these goings-on. Women have book clubs, hobby groups, coffee clubs and fund-raising movie nights.

I'm all for these events if you enjoy them, but even then: how many activities can you fit in before they start to detract from your quality of life rather than add to it?

The usual greeting of 'Hi, how are you? How have you been lately?' is usually responded to with a 'Good thanks, busy as always; I've got so much on you wouldn't believe'. I've even heard that 'Busy, busy!' has replaced 'Fine thanks' as a standard response to 'How are you?'

Imagine if instead of detailing how busy you are, you responded 'Great thanks. I've got tons of free time and I've completed my to-do list for the month. Life is really cruisy and I plan to read a book this afternoon.' People would stare at you and probably not know what to say, because it seems to be more socially acceptable to be busy and stressed than living a streamlined life of rest and relaxation.

The bliss of a life with space in it

Imagine if you really did have a life full of ease, with time to relax and minimal stress. Do you think you would be in better health? Imagine if you prepared meals ahead of time and ate well so that you were slender in a seemingly effortless way. Wouldn't that be wonderful?

But why should it be a pipe dream? If you want to live a long and healthy life and actually enjoy your life, it's imperative that you streamline your days as much as possible, as well as create a mindset of ease. There are a small percentage of people who thrive on being flat-out and full-on all the time, but for most of us it's detrimental to our wellbeing.

Being over-busy is making us fat

When we pack too much into every single day we are stressing ourselves in little ways, all of the time. When we are stressed, we eat; it's a response directed by nature. Stress hormones make us want to eat, preferably simple carbohydrates and processed foods, to calm us with the soothing effects they provide.

Problems arising from a busy lifestyle include:

We are too tired to prepare food so we buy takeout or boxed supermarket foods to create all or part of our meals. We don't have time to plan ahead for our meals which means we choose a quick and easy – but not necessarily healthy – option.

We feel tired, so pick up a sweet treat for an energy boost or to give ourselves a minute to relax.

We feel like we are looking after everyone but ourselves so we treat ourselves with something yummy and decadent as a reward or consolation (for me it is sugary sweets and chocolate – I can inhale them and I swear I am not overstating that).

We feel resentful that we're the one doing everything, which also triggers comfort eating.

Often we will simply accept that life is busy, hard, and a struggle to keep on top of. It's rare that we would stop and think – *How can I simplify, streamline and organize myself better for a more efficient life full of ease?* A simpler life doesn't just happen; it needs intentional thought.

Having a simpler, easier life is simultaneously a practical and a mindset issue

Practically speaking, it's about setting yourself up for success by creating routines that flow and bring ease into your day. As far as mindset goes, it's about giving yourself permission to have an easier life and letting go of the guilt that you might experience from desiring this.

One benefit of allowing more space to exist in your life is having time to shop for and prepare meals. Traditionally, Europeans will shop daily for food provisions and make meal preparation an important part of their day. You may not want to go this far but it's a good thing to keep in mind.

My favourite healthy lunch is a big salad with plenty of protein and a delicious dressing. When I have time to wash, peel and slice vegetables, and I've cooked some chicken the night before to shred on top, it's a pleasure to make my salad. I put some music or a podcast on and get chopping.

Conversely, when I have no time, it's a chore which I put off, half do or even end up flagging and buying a less healthy (and more expensive) lunch instead.

The other question to consider is, *Am I allowing myself to have an easier life and if not, why not?* Where did we learn that it is selfish and uncaring to want to enjoy life and have time to rest and relax without judgement from others? Is it that we feel we are lazy if we don't fill every minute of every day with tasks and to-dos?

Imagine a life where you have time to do everything you must do, the things you want to do, and time to rest and rejuvenate as well. A life where you have margin between activities – space to breathe.

When you feel calm and productive, you eat better, you rest better, and you have time for a little bit of exercise each day. Simply put, your health will be improved and you are likely to be slimmer.

Structuring for an easier life

If you let yourself have an easier life and set up your plans around that, you will set yourself up for success. It means that you look at what you have on and think:

How can I make it easier?

Can I delete it? Do I even want to keep it in my life?

What are my top priorities and what can I put at the bottom of the list?

This is not about doing nothing; rather, it is prioritising what is important to you and letting the other obligations slide away, without guilt. And it can be big or small parts of your life.

Simplifying around your job or career

A big change might mean looking at your job with a long commute each way. Can you apply for a position closer to home? Can you ask your employers if your role can be made into a four-day-a-week job instead? Or, can your job be made part-time or job-shared so you can work three days a week rather than five?

Here's a suggestion you might find extreme – can you move closer to your job? It might sound over-the-top but why not consider everything. A commute is a big part of your life and can add stress as well as draining your energy.

I know mothers who work four days a week, and for the one day when their husband is at work and their children are at school or in day-care, they get to catch up on housework, do grocery shopping, have appointments and take care of the running of the household so that they can enjoy the weekend with their family.

Plus there are enjoyable tasks such as getting your hair done, having a manicure or massage and being creative at home. One day a week where you can have your own space and feel relaxed. It might mean you go to a movie, or you may go for a long walk. Have it feel open and free, and you will find yourself making healthier choices.

Think of this extra day as breathing space. Ask yourself, is that something that would be beneficial to you?

You might think, *I need the money, Fiona, everyone does*, and of course you do, that's definitely a major consideration; but you might work out that you actually spend money on things you wouldn't have to if you had more time at home.

You might spend money on stuff to make yourself feel better than if you had more down-time. Having one day a week entirely to yourself – imagine that! – maybe then you wouldn't feel compelled to fill yourself up with shopping.

But it feels selfish; you should save those days off for a family vacation; you should use that day to help someone out; you should use it to declutter the garage. You need to stop those martyr thoughts in their tracks; they are what landed you in this mess in the first place.

If you do take a day off work, whether it's a new ongoing thing, or booking in an extra day's leave every once in a while, consider not telling anyone outside of your household. When you have time, other people can think it's their right to use it up.

Imagine how blissful it would be to book one day's leave from work on a regular basis, perhaps every two or three months, where you do exactly what *you* want.

In the end, it's all about giving yourself permission – permission to enjoy your life! When we feel like we are putting ourselves last all the time, we often rebel in our own ways (I know I do) and eat our favourite treat foods for comfort, no matter how unhappy they make us afterwards.

Be strong in your decision

There is a real, physical detriment from being too busy. When we have a lot to do, we may go to bed later because we are trying to fit everything in. This can make our body hold onto fat (there are many studies which show the later you go to bed on a consistent basis, the fatter you are likely to be).

Other people might not approve of you making your life easier and it could even be those closest to you. It's not because you are leaning on them or making them do more of the work; it's because they can see you enjoying your life as well as making progress. They may think, perhaps subconsciously, *Well I'm busy, so you should be too.*

I've seen many people wear busyness like a badge of honour and it seems like they want to make you feel bad for your relaxed happiness. You're driving home and dinner is all organized. As you head off to bed to read about 9pm, you feel a sense of guilt as you remember how they told you they are up past midnight every night just to get everything done.

I used to feel like I should be doing more too, but I have gained strength in owning my choices now and I don't feel that way anymore. I am structuring my life the way I want to live it. I want my days to feel free, relaxed and happy. I want time to decompress in between jobs, errands, hobbies and family.

And I wonder, how much of that needs to be done and how much is busy-work?

Ask yourself 'How quickly can I do this?'

I used to see it when we owned a shoe store – a customer would come in for a pair of shoes and they'd already been around six shoe shops. They'd tell me they've not been able to find exactly the pair they have in mind and fair enough, if there is a specific dress colour to match, I get it. But these people only wanted a casual pair of shoes for the weekend and they were making it into such a big time-sucking ordeal for themselves.

When I go shopping, I try to make decisions as quickly as possible. Sometimes it's nice to browse to see what is new for the season, but mostly I find that quite boring if I don't need to buy anything.

I don't like to spend a whole day going around the shops to choose a top, for example. When I bought a new winter sweater recently, I chose a particular store to start with. I liked their styles and the prices were good. I found a few options there so I bought them and carried on with my life. I didn't need to research every top available in every store.

I know we are all different in how we like to approach shopping, but for me I would rather simplify my life and not spend it rushing around packing a lot into it. Shopping is only one example of how I like to minimise time spent without sacrificing my quality of decision-making.

Let more space into your life

I don't have a lot of obligations for clubs and activities because I value unstructured time. I do often pack a lot into one day, but it's all on my terms and includes time to rest, recharge and relax. I read, cook, watch television (usually one episode of my current program each night), talk to my husband, write, clean, organize our home and exercise.

Most of these activities can be done in my own time and when I want to do them. That means I am in charge, which feels better than always needing to watch the clock because you have something on every day.

How this relates to your weight is that when you are always on the go and busy; even if it was originally of your own making, you start feeling under the gun and like you never have a moment to yourself. Then you look for a pleasurable release; you eat something as an excuse to take a break, or you treat yourself because you're feeling so run down.

The stress of always being busy, even a small, manageable amount of busy is quite hard on your health. Your cortisol levels are permanently raised and your fight or flight response is elevated, which drains your adrenalin instead of keeping it for a true emergency. All of this makes you crave high-sugar, high-carbohydrate processed foods and causes you to store fat around your stomach.

Being too busy all the time is *really* bad for your health

It's this diminishing circle of unhealthiness and unhappiness that we are creating by not letting ourselves have what we would consider an easy life; to do a reasonable number of tasks in a day and an appropriate day's work.

Writing this chapter is hyping me up and not in a good way. It shows you the power of words, even if you say them as a joke or to blend in when you are making small talk. I am going to challenge myself not to use the word busy. It rolls off the tongue, doesn't it? How about rewording it differently – if someone asks how work is, say 'it's going great thanks' instead of 'we're crazy busy at the moment, as usual'. It has a more relaxed feeling.

Go through your diary or planner and see all the tasks that you do. Write them all down on a big list. Then think about your life and every task, routine and activity you do on a daily basis. There will be entries on this list which drain you.

Some of the items on your list will be non-negotiables. You might not want to get rid of your husband and children, for example. You might be responsible for an elderly or sick parent. You don't want to change your job situation.

Tick the items that are non-negotiable – such as your family – and tick the items you love doing, then look at the rest. You might not quit something completely, but even taking a season off if you feel you need to create some breathing space in your schedule can be helpful. You will then get a chance to see if you miss it or not.

If it's a book club that has become more of an obligation than a joy, let it go. People probably won't be happy that you are 'quitting', so you will need to be polite yet firm, and remember why you are doing it. Let them know that you won't be able to attend book club any more.

For four years I volunteered at the SPCA once a month on a Sunday morning. When my husband and I opened our shoe store we started out working six days a week. At that time I gave notice to my team leader that I could no longer volunteer.

Instead of the 'Thanks and good luck' I was expecting to receive, she was very upset with me and quite unpleasant. She asked why I couldn't still work Sundays because our store was open Monday to Saturday.

I would have loved to have stayed helping out because I really enjoyed the work, but I could see they had plenty of good quality, long-term volunteers and I now only had four days off per month to do my chores and have a life. I could have gone back on my decision, but I held firm. I needed to open up some space.

Open up space for peace and happiness

Remember, when you are feeling too bogged down with your life, you eat for pleasure and to escape. You are actively changing that dynamic now, and it may feel uncomfortable. This is because you are moving outside of your comfort zone (that's literally the discomfort) with the things you are doing – deciding what *you* want, letting people know how it's going to be from now on and putting boundaries into place.

Having time to go for a walk, read a book, watch a television program or play around with your hobbies makes you feel happy and content, and you are less like to binge on temporary feel-good carbs to get that same happy feeling.

Having time for a face mask, putting on foot cream or whatever makes you feel good means you are happy with an herbal tea after dinner instead of eating two (or three, it's been done before) bowls of ice-cream.

It simply requires a little bit of rewiring, and letting go of the guilt that heaven forbid, you should relax and enjoy your life.

Your *Thirty Slim Days* action tips:

Look at your weekly schedule as if with someone else's eyes. Would they think it was reasonable? What would they say if you asked them what you could change or leave out?

If I asked you what you really dislike in your schedule, what pops out for you straight away? Is it a school or volunteer position? Maybe it's your job. Can you delete or change these things?

Start to tell yourself:
It's okay to rest
I don't have to work all hours of the day
Others can do their bit too
It's okay to ask for help

Set reasonable sleep and wake times and stick to them, even if there are tasks you think you need to do. If you've been busy all day and still have jobs to do at 11pm, chances are you are packing too much in.

If you have been dawdling around and then suddenly find yourself needing to finish jobs late at night, this could be a sign that you need to manage your time better. This is what I used do all the time. I don't do it every day now, but I sometimes write a to-do list in the morning and check back to it often as I work through the items. It's amazing how much I get done on those days – who would've thought!

Day 14
Who are you going to feed?

If you are anything like me, there are two distinct sides to you.

Firstly, there is the person who desires to be slim and healthy. This gorgeous person looks amazing in her chic outfits and wears everything in her wardrobe on a regular basis. There are no skinny clothes pushed down to the end of the rail. She knows that she wants to be slender and vibrant and eats (and drinks) accordingly.

Then there is the person who eats what she wants at any old time. She doesn't deny herself any of the treat foods that she loves. If she has a craving, she satisfies it. She hates that she can't fit her lovely clothes but she can't see herself giving up all those little treats that make life more pleasurable.

I wish I was the first person and on brief occasions I have been; but the truth is I was more often the second person. However, that will not stop me striving to be the first person.

I always felt like I was denying myself of pleasure and depriving myself of a good time when I did not have fun foods in my diet. Even though I love healthy fresh fruits and vegetables, eggs, lean meats and fish, raw nuts and lots of cool, clear water to drink; I don't consider these foods fun. Healthy and nourishing – yes, fun – no.

With no treat foods in my life it seemed a bleak existence, like those movies where they tint the film grey to show how grim life is for the characters portrayed. I didn't want to live in that movie, I wanted to live in the colourful one filled with bright and cheery treat foods.

This has always been my main stumbling block in living a slender, chic and healthy life. I've been torn between my two favoured worlds and I couldn't have it both ways because they were mutually exclusive.

My solution over the years was to eat healthy at my three meals a day most of the time, but still have snack foods in between. This meant I was always heavier than I would have liked to be, and felt frumpy in my clothes. There were also many clothes that were simply too tight to be worn, and they mocked me from my closet.

Yes, the fun side of me won out most of the time, but it wasn't fun feeling blobby.

Food as an addiction?

In her excellent book *Eating Less: Say goodbye to overeating* by Gillian Riley, she talks about food being addictive and many of us being addicted to certain types of food. According to Gillian, you can be underweight, a normal weight or overweight and still be a food addict.

Those with a lower weight might eat smaller portions of the addictive foods, but for most people, their addiction for certain foods shows up on their body as excess weight.

In addition, Gillian says there are degrees of food addiction.

Going through her long list of addictive characteristics in the book, I realized I said *Yes* to all of them except one (which was about not getting your five-plus a day of fresh fruits and vegetables). Here are a few from the list:

- *Being obsessed with food*
- *Not feeling satisfied with small portions*
- *Despite certain foods detracting from your health, you still eat them*
- *Finding it challenging to stick to a diet*
- *Regaining weight lost again*
- *Thinking about food much of the time*
- *Feeling hungry much of the time*
- *Regularly feeling regretful of how much or what you have eaten*

- *Consistently making and breaking promises to yourself about what you will and won't eat*

May I repeat: I said *Yes* to twenty out of the twenty-one items. What an eye-opener that was.

I didn't want to be an addict, but there was a part of me who was – around food. Apart from thinking to myself, *I don't want to be called an addict*; I then realized what an amazing opportunity this was.

You can't reason with an addict. You can't offer the choice to an addict because they will always take the addict's choice – more of their favoured drug. You can't trust an addict; they are sneaky and will let you down every time.

You may not like calling yourself an addict, and I don't either, but in actual fact it is the food that is addictive. Those faux foods which are designed to be highly addictive to humans. The salt, fat, wheat and sugar sets off pleasure sensors in the brain which are much like those that are pushed when someone takes recreational drugs.

Once you have one, you want another. I ask you; have you ever had 'just one' potato chip? Or 'just one' bite of chocolate?

The trick is not to let the addict get that taste in the first place.

Saying to myself whenever I was faced with a choice between buying the cheap and crappy snack food or being chic and sticking to my three meals a day plan: *'Are you going to listen to the slim and elegant you?*

Or are you going to listen to the addict?', it was an *easy* decision to say 'No'.

No, I am not going to give in to the addict.
No, I am not going to support the addict.
No, I am not going to listen to the addict.

It sounds harsh to talk about being addicted, but it is so much easier to make good food choices when I choose to listen to my higher self – the chic and slender lady of my dreams; instead of listening to a person who cannot be trusted and only wants to satisfy their cravings.

The one you feed

There is a parable which you may have heard of, called *'The One You Feed'*. If you haven't heard this parable, I'll share it briefly:

A grandfather was talking with his grandson. He tells him that there are two wolves fighting inside us (which explains our inner conflicts).

One of them is a good wolf which represents such attributes as light, hope, kindness, bravery and love. The other is a bad wolf, which represents despair, greed, darkness, hatred and fear.

The grandson stops and thinks about it for a second, then looks up at his grandfather and asks, "Grandfather, which one wins?"

The grandfather quietly replies, "The one you choose to feed".

This parable came to mind when I was writing this chapter, and the concept of which side of yourself you should choose to give your attention, time and trust to. In this case, the parable asks which side of you are you going to (literally) feed and therefore strengthen?

It struck me that it could be thought about exactly the same if you are trying to save money to pay off debt and get ahead, but you are always tempted by shop sales and buying yourself something new, bright and shiny.

Which one of you are you going to give your credit card to?

The you who desires to be savvy and financially smart, who always pays her bills on time and has money in the bank?

Or the shyster you, who would steal your money as soon as your back was turned, and run up debts then skip town? The one who is addicted to shopping despite knowing how it lands her in more debt?

Which one would you trust with your PIN number?

Rephrase your innocent enough thought that it would be nice to go out and have a browse at the mall or an ice-cream because it's summery. Strengthen the side of you who is your best self. Turn away from the other part of you who only wants to satisfy her base levels and doesn't care about your future.

This is how I found it almost instantly easy to say *No* to the foods that had caused me so much misery over the years. Happiness at the time, but misery afterwards as I had broken yet another promise to myself.

My husband says something that always makes me laugh, and it is this:

No-one ever wakes up in the morning wishing they had eaten an entire king-size bar of dairy milk chocolate the night before.

You might want that giant-size chocolate bar after dinner, but when you wake up in the morning, you won't wish that. You will be glad you didn't have it.

Imagine waking up saying 'Gee, I'm really glad I gorged myself last night'. No-one ever says that, do they! No, it's more the regret of stuffing yourself and resolving not to do it again... until the next time.

Asking yourself this simple question:

Am I going to listen to my slim and elegant self?
Or am I going to listen to the addict?

...is all you need to turn around an iffy situation. It's that easy.

Accept that there are some foods that might never agree with you

There are people around who can take or leave any food, treating it as mere fuel for the body and don't look upon food and eating as a pleasurable pastime. But for most of us, we derive immense pleasure from eating, sometimes too much.

If you are like me, it's not all foods that cause your mind to tip upside down and lose self-control though. It's not like I have to portion out fruit and vegetables and tell myself not to eat too much of them.

I have already realized that with normal, real whole foods, my body and mind knows what to do with them and doesn't have an issue with over-consuming them.

No, it's the processed un-real snack foods that cause me the problems, and that's because junk food is produced to be addictive. Salt, sugar, wheat, fat; these are the addictive substances – some even believe sugar to be more addictive than cocaine.

Those sneaky (and rich) processed food corporations know they can make a fortune producing cheap-to-make addictive substances which customers flock to. It's almost criminal when you think about it, especially when they start their consumers off as children, marketing these foods as a fun treat. They are neither fun nor a treat for our bodies.

I found it an easy to know what foods were addictable to me. I divided foods up into what I could eat in a normal way and what I couldn't – those foods that I simply could not go easy on once I'd started or which caused cravings in me.

I then knew which were the addictive foods and could put them into the '*I don't want you in my life*' category. For an extra safeguard I apply the addict question to them if temptation arises.

For me, those foods are:

Potato chips
Corn chips
Roasted and salted nuts
Sweet fizzy drinks (diet/non-diet)
Lollies/sweets/candy
Marshmallows
Milk chocolate, white chocolate
Ice-cream
Popcorn
Licorice

Now, take a look at that list. Is there anything fresh and healthy on that list? Or is it mostly a bunch of processed carbohydrates with zero nutritional value?

For you it may be a similar list, or you may have different entries on yours. I'm not really fussed about biscuits (cookies), pie or bread, but I know these are huge obstacles for others.

For my husband, he doesn't find my list appealing at all; he much prefers savoury items and keeps well away from meat pies and hamburgers because he knows they could be his downfall if he let them be.

Brainstorming my list, there is now a clear-cut line that I can draw when a tiny voice in my head says, *Let's go get something fun to eat – you haven't had kettle corn in a while.*

You already know what I am going to say to myself – '*Am I going to listen to the addict?*'

Your *Thirty Slim Days* action tips:

Write down all the foods that you have a **love/hate relationship** with. Foods that you wished did not exist, because then you would not have to deal with them.

Note down your most adored snack foods and everything you cannot say no to, but which make you **unhappy after you have eaten them**, either with an upset tummy or gaining weight.

You now have your list. Next time you want to eat one of those foods, ask yourself:

'*Am I going to listen to the addict?*'

Day 15
Choose small, daily body movement

I am naturally a person who prefers to relax and read than go for a run. I don't like to say sloth-like, because I am choosing to speak kindly to myself now; however I do love to feel comfortable, and exercise usually isn't that comfortable.

Exercise is something that many of us avoid. I know I did for a long time and I still don't really like structured, formal or group exercise. Yes... I am an introvert. For extroverts or 'people' people, you may love the social contact and accountability that a group class or exercise club gives you. For others, we could think of nothing worse!

The most important thing about exercise is to find something you enjoy doing, then you won't mind doing it. Call me crazy, but you might even find yourself looking forward to it.

For me, I love to go for a walk. I can do it at any time of the day (although I prefer to do it in the morning if possible), it's free and it gets me out into nature and exposure to a bit of Vitamin D.

In the back of my mind I've always known that I 'should' be doing more weight-bearing exercise, especially being a woman going into *a certain age*. Weight-bearing exercise or resistance training as it's also known helps prevent osteoporosis and I'm sure a whole host of getting-older maladies if I wanted to google a list.

Making the right thing to do an easy choice

In addition, doing weights helps with being slim, because having slightly more muscle on your body means you are burning fat, even if you are sitting on the sofa because muscle uses fat for energy.

Despite knowing all this, I still did not do any resistance training at all. At least I'm walking, I would tell myself. But some days I wouldn't even do that.

Recently I was listening to a radio interview about this very topic – how a weight-bearing workout is so important for women – right before I headed out for a walk. I was in my leggings and tee-shirt with running shoes on. I planned to go on a route that took about forty-five minutes.

I locked the front door and saw there was a very fine drizzly but persistent rain. I don't mind if it spits on me a little bit when I'm already on a walk, but I won't go if it looks like imminent rain, and I definitely do not go if it's already raining.

Feeling a little bit silly, I turned around on the driveway and walked back to our front door, letting myself in again.

In this moment, I decided that both the radio interview lady and the rain was a sign from the universe that I should try a weight-bearing workout. I've always wanted to be motivated enough to do indoor workouts but never have. There are unused DVDs and a very new looking yoga mat (even though I've had it for a number of years) at my house.

In my inspiration files, I have a small 'Slimming and Health' folder of torn-out pages, so I opened that and chose a simple workout from a woman's magazine. Over the next fifteen minutes I did:

20 lunges (ten on each side) – take a big step back and dip down, then up. Swap to the other side and repeat.

20 t-birds – stand up straight, letting your arms hang down. Turn your thumbs out and raise your arms to create a t-shape. At the same time squat down. Squeeze your shoulder blades together and engage your core (stomach) area. Hold this pose or raise your arms up and down (small circles are good too). Arms down, stand up straight and repeat.

20 press-ups – against the kitchen counter. You can do them in a door frame too, it's an excellent, easier, way to start than on the ground.

20 step-ups (ten on each side) – we have a two-storey house so I did them on our stairs (covering two stairs with each step).

20 squat salutations – drop into a half-squat. Shoot your hips forward and raise your arms to stand, firming all your muscles. Arms down and repeat.

20 single leg lowerings (ten on each side) – lie down with arms beside you (I was pleased to use my yoga mat, see, it wasn't a waste of money!) Pull your belly button into your spine and alternate lifting one leg up.

10 sit ups – I didn't think I would make it to twenty, so I did ten. I lay on the yoga mat, with knees bent and lifted myself up and down slowly, with arms by my side lifting too.

Then, I finished doing some stretches that felt good on my pristine yoga mat for a few minutes.

I looked at the clock when I'd finished and all up my workout took me fifteen minutes. In the past, I would have decided a fifteen-minute workout wasn't worth the effort, but judging by how I felt the next day – I had quite a few sore muscles, but not too sore – it definitely was.

I began to see that small amounts were the key, and I have been applying this to my walks too. Instead of thinking to myself 'it's an hour or it's not worth going', I often skipped it if I felt like I didn't have the energy for an hour. Now, it's twenty to forty-five minutes. Even if it's *ten minutes*, at least I'm getting my blood moving and loosening up my joints and muscles.

Removing excuses

In the past I also used the justification that I had no equipment to do a weight-bearing workout at home; I'd need to go buy some proper equipment. Wrong! I had the perfect piece of equipment right here with me at home – my body.

Simple google 'hotel room workout' (doing this on YouTube is good because then you get a moving visual of how an exercise is supposed to look) and see what an easy, free-of-cost and instant workout looks like.

I'm not perfect here, I was enthused about a free, at-home workout for quite a few months before I actually did one. And now that I have, I know they are a good idea. Not only a good idea, but I look forward to them.

One big drawcard is the brevity. I can do a fifteen-minute workout and be done for the day. Sure, proper gym people might not think it's enough, but that's okay, I'm not asking them to do this workout. I'm finding a workout that's right for me, and if it's one I will actually do, I'm on a winner.

My plan is to alternate a walk one day with my fifteen-minute weight bearing workout the next, three times a week each.

It would work well with yoga too, because the Iyengar Yoga classes I go to on-and-off were definitely weight bearing. I used to have sore muscles the day after a class. Having been to a few classes was very useful in knowing how to do the exercises myself at home, because then I knew the correct way to do them.

So if I wanted a change from my resistance training, I could do a petite yoga workout instead. Or spring for a class.

Just do fifteen minutes

On days when you can't be bothered with even fifteen minutes – consider this. Once you get started, your little workout can be pleasant and enjoyable, and you will definitely feel good afterwards – far better than if you hadn't bothered, both physically and also with the satisfaction of doing what you said you were going to do.

Over time, these fifteen-minute periods of movement will add up to better health and mobility. Think of it like brushing your teeth. You probably wouldn't see a decline in the state of your teeth from skipping a day, however imagine going years without brushing your teeth. It wouldn't be good!

It's the same with movement. Many of us spend so long sitting at a desk or in a car that it can feel like our body is in the seated position for much of our day. Imagine you are your body; I know you *are* your body, but think from the point of view of your body – it will be saying to you, *I feel stiff, please move me around.*

So how can you change your mindset around movement from 'Urgh, can't be bothered' to 'yay!' Here are my tips on setting up a supportive environment:

Book in a minimum as a non-negotiable – as early in the day as you can, or at a time when you know you will do it. Look at your planner and schedule in when you are doing to do three fifteen-minute weight workouts over the next week, and when you are going to do two or three walks.

Make sure you have good gear – if you want to wear exercise clothing, get yourself a couple of sets. If you choose to wear your normal clothes, sort out a pair of comfortable shoes. Always have everything clean and ready to go.

Finding time in your work day

It can be hard when you are working full-time. I know there were many days where there wasn't enough time in the morning, and it was too late when I arrived home because I had to cook dinner straight away or it was already dark.

On those days, I'd go for a ten- or fifteen-minute walk around the block from work in my lunch break. It was a nice change from being under fluorescent lights. If the clouds looked threatening I'd take a fold-up umbrella.

Maybe there wasn't even time for a walk at lunchtime, perhaps you had errands to do and lunch to eat. Something that is fun is do, is turn on the music and do your own one-song workout while dinner is cooking. You can dance or do what I do – my own nineties-style aerobics class where I spring around like a loon – no-one else is there so it's okay! Do you remember how to do the grapevine?

I also find this is a good warm-up act before my at-home workout. Choose a song that has a steady pace and also make it one that you love. One song is quite long when you are moving non-stop and it really elevates the heart rate. Remember, don't stop until the song has finished.

One of my very favourites for doing this is 'Suddenly I See' by KT Tunstall. It is the opening song to the movie 'The Devil Wears Prada' and if you search for that on YouTube you not only get to listen to the song, but you also can view a very inspiring montage of slim, stylish New York City women getting ready for their day.

Be your own cheerleader

To head off the 'can't be bothered' feeling you are likely to encounter at some stage, consider all the reasons why doing small amounts of movement is a good idea so you will have a list to refer to at those times. For me:

- I will feel good afterwards
- It's a loving thing to do for my body
- I will feel better about myself and have higher self-esteem
- I will have time to think by myself
- I can listen to music, podcasts or audiobooks
- I will sleep better
- I will have more energy
- I will gain strength and flexibility
- My muscles will become more toned over time
- Weight maintenance will be easier as I age
- I will be one of those fit older people one day
- It will become a habit; then I won't have to decide whether I want to do it or not
- I love being out in nature when I go for a walk (even if it's streets and houses rather than a peaceful bushwalk)
- I feel good after a resistance-training workout – I can feel my muscles

What your body looks and feels like today is a result of how much and what kind of exercise you have done in the past. Don't feel demoralized if you do one day's fifteen-minute workout and think 'it's no use'.

Imagine yourself six months into the future, even two years or five years, having done a small exercise routine each day. Thirty-minutes' walk every second day, with ten sit-ups and twenty doorframe push-ups on the alternating days doesn't sound like much, but it all adds up.

When they are that small and doable, they will become as routine to you as making the bed. Sure you can do more if you want, but get that solid baseline of fifteen minutes a day to start with. You can do it!

Your *Thirty Slim Days* action tips:

Make a decision. Decide that from today on you will move your body with intention, even if it's for only five minutes a day.

Get into the routine of doing something that **feels good to your body** (not to your *mind*, to your body – your mind will say 'no, let's go do something more fun!').

Research 'hotel room workout' on YouTube to **get some ideas on at-home workouts** that require no equipment. Most of them are short – about ten minutes – and you can follow along.

Note down ideas to **make movement fun**. Have this list to hand and choose one each day – make sure you do resistance training three times a week; don't only do cardio. Resistance training is good for burning fat, strengthening your bones and toning muscle.

Think outside the box when it comes to mini-workouts. I've always loved the sensuality of Latin dance, but have never gone to a lesson. Searching for 'beginners tango workout' on YouTube brought up a number of different video classes which would be a fun workout at home.

Reframe your thoughts: Instead of hating your body, do something because you *love* your body (I'm talking about deep down unconditional love like you would have for a family member, not loving that your thighs have started rubbing together).

Instead of thinking to yourself 'I have to exercise because I hate my body and want to change it', think 'I'm going to exercise today because **I love my body** and want her to be healthy and happy'.

Day 16
Visit your future self

Mindset is a huge part of being slim. It's so hard to do something when you have to, and so effortless when you want to. That's my goal with everything I want to do in life, from eating healthy, to exercising, keeping my home clean and clutter-free and writing my books. I find ways to make the right thing to do *effortless*.

To get started on the best path I find it helps to have inspiration to motivate me.

You would think an end result of looking great in your clothes and feeling amazingly healthy and vibrant would be enough of a motivation; apparently not though, otherwise none of us would give food a second thought between our healthy and balanced meals.

Having your own well of inspiration that you are constantly topping up from is crucial to keeping you on track so that you can easily become – and stay at – your happy weight.

Welcome! Come on in!

A fun way to self-inspire is by visiting your future self. The basic premise is that you visit your ideal self in the future and ask her how she did it.

Choose a timeframe that feels good to you; it might be different at different times. For example, you might choose to look six months into the future, or imagine yourself on your next birthday. Maybe it's five or ten years' time, or even the retirement you. I love to visit the retirement me – she's awesome.

You can choose to visit the future you that carries on with the same habits and choices you are making now, or instead you can call upon the future you who embodies everything you dream of – good health, consistent slimness, beauty, style, financial success and happiness.

I'm sure you can guess which one is going to be more inspiring – that's right: the happy, healthy and successful you.

While you are visiting your amazing self in the future, observe all the details of your dream life. Everything you desire and more, she already has it. She is content and happy and it shows.

What does she look like?

How does her hair look – the colour, style, condition of it?

What does her face look like? What does the face of someone who has been living a healthy and fun dream life look like?

Is she slim and vibrant?

Is her stance confident and friendly?

What is she wearing? Describe her outfit.

What colours does she wear?

What kind of a house does she live in? Is it a French-style stone home? A cottage in the country? An apartment in the city?

Imagine you are going to visit her. Go up to her home and knock on the front door. When she answers, let her take you inside for a look around. See how your future self has decorated her home; see how it is exquisite and exactly to your taste.

Walk into her bedroom. It is beautiful – a sanctuary – and you are excited to see the perfect closet and ensuite bathroom for you. What does the master bedroom look like? Describe the décor and take notice of the details.

Next you go into the kitchen and see how she has set herself up to be a slim and healthy success. What do the pantry shelves contain? Open her fridge and see what is inside. She won't mind.

There is one more room to look at – off the living room there is a nook. What is in there? Is it a library or office? A sewing or craft room? This is your future self's own private space where she goes to relax and create. Note what you see in there. Be inspired that she takes time out for herself to rejuvenate.

See how healthy and happy she looks – she absolutely glows! Ask her:

What you have done to gain the results you have now?
What has been the single most important thing you would recommend I do right now?
What advice do you have for me?
What were some of the big changes you had to make?
What is your biggest tip for success?
Where should I go from here?
How did you create this life?
What was your biggest challenge?
How did you become so slim and healthy and be consistent about it?

You don't have to answer every single question at once or even in depth. You could choose one to focus on in a single sitting. I asked my future self, as a slim and healthy person who has been that way for many years, how she created this way of life and she told me:

- I trained myself into enjoying healthy foods and out of unhealthy snack foods – I reverse brainwashed myself

- I gave up the notion of scheduled exercise and instead made activity and movement a part of my day
- I enjoy stretches every night before bed
- I keep good wake and sleep hours
- I built good routines into my life that made the healthy option the default
- I streamlined and decluttered my kitchen, my closet and my whole home and kept it that way – it helps me to feel light which flows through to my food choices
- I indulge in activities I enjoy such as reading, watching movies, going out for coffee and day-trips, and crafts – that way I don't look to food to bring pleasure into my life
- I surround myself with simple luxury and home comforts, with plenty of non-food pleasures
- I addressed foods that I couldn't eat normally and eliminated them from my life completely, after realizing that anything I ate in an addictive way was trying to tell me they were not my food
- I made decisions about what I would and wouldn't do and drew them up as guidelines for how I wanted to live my life
- I remembered I am slim, elegant, serene and stylish, every single day and ate, groomed and carried myself accordingly

- I no longer listened to that sabotaging voice in my head that told me 'one won't hurt' when I knew from previous experience that that was not true
- I created a healthy eating plan for myself and followed through, regardless of whether I felt like it or not
- I started to look at food as a pleasurable fuel rather than a way to soothe my emotions as I had done in the past
- I ate *more* food – more fruit, more fresh vegetables, more herbal teas, more water, more lean protein at meals
- I eat three meals a day and do not snack – it was hard to start with but then I became used to it and now I don't even think about it

Wow, all of this came from me, and I now have an extremely motivating blueprint for how to get me to that slim and healthy future self, in a fun and enjoyable way. I am always astounded at what I come up with, and I think you will be too if you ask your future self. She'd be thrilled to hear from you.

The magazine interview technique

Another future self exercise I love to practice is the magazine interview technique.

Fast forward into the future when you have your dream perfect figure. You are being interviewed by a magazine and they want to know all of your weight loss secrets. They say to you, 'You look so amazing! You've lost an incredible amount of weight. You look happy, and you've kept it off a long time now. Please tell us your secrets to weight loss success'.

You are answering your interviewer as your future self, the 2.0 version. Step forward as the person you imagine yourself as and answer them from there. You have reached your goal weight and stayed there for a number of years now. You are answering your interviewer as that person who looks and feels fantastic, who lives her life in a way that supports a healthy and slender figure.

It may sound a little silly to you, but when I've done this exercise, I have been amazed at what comes out – and it's come from my mind, not something I have copied. So it really is within me, I realized.

It's much easier to answer than if I asked myself, *What do I have to do to lose weight?* But it gives you the same answers.

When I am 'interviewed', it might go like this:

Fiona, you've dropped an incredible amount of weight over the past six months. How much have you lost and how did you do it? We're all dying to know.

'Hi, thanks so much and yes, I am very proud of how I look now. It's like night and day to how I was before. I lost about thirteen kilos and now weigh 61kg. How

did I do it? I chose to be smoking hot and sexy at forty-six and carried on from there, really!

I decided that I loved being disciplined and strict and enjoyed seeing the weight peel off me. I actually lost the first ten kilos in three months and then gradually the last few came off as well. I am in the best shape I've ever been in and I'm loving my new lease of life. I look and feel ten years younger and love getting dressed in the morning now.

I had already cut out wheat and other gluten-containing foods because I was diagnosed celiac a number of years ago. I also found that dairy made my tummy unhappy so I cut most of that out too, plus sugar. Sugar was my biggest problem, but once I made the decision to be the person I've always wanted to be – focused, disciplined, successful and in incredible shape, it was easy to say no to those foods. They just didn't interest me anymore.

I used to not be able to go a day without lollies and chocolate and if I lasted a week it was a miracle. These days I don't even think about those foods and instead enjoy nourishing my body with lean meat, fish, eggs, fresh fruit, fresh vegetables and raw nuts. Plenty of water too – I drink water all day long and if I want a hot drink I'll have an herbal or green tea with the occasional soy latte.

I suppose paleo is the best way to describe my eating style, I find it suits me best. It keeps me full between meals and it's natural and healthy.'

And here's another I wrote for myself, before I lost any weight, but imagining myself as that future person who didn't have issues with her weight and eating.

Fiona, what's it like being skinny?

'I love being thin because I feel confident and happy with myself. I feel in control and know that people aren't looking at me and judging me for being overweight (they must do that because I used to do it to others).

I love fitting into all of my clothes and looking amazing in them. I love my skinny shoulders and flat stomach. I love not having a pudgy overhang on my jeans waistband. I love having smaller boobs and a defined jawline. I love that my skin looks glowing and healthy from nutritious food.

I love not dieting and instead eating food that is good for me. I love not being beholden to sugar and refined carbs. I simply don't eat them anymore and don't miss them. The thought of eating something is ALWAYS better than the reality.

I also feel a lot sexier when I'm thin. Being fatter really kills the libido. And I love that my husband is attracted to me more. He can't help it, men are visual creatures and will notice a beautiful, slim woman who takes care of herself. I can't get enough of myself and I know my husband feels the same.'

Some of these statements were true and what I did already, and some were not true at the time. By mixing in truth and what I wished was true, it brought the whole picture closer to me.

Your mind doesn't know the difference between fact and fiction, so you can use it to your advantage.

What is so powerful about this technique is that you are digging answers out of yourself and it's coming from within you. If you asked yourself this question differently you might be stumped. But by asking 'what are the secrets to your success' you are zooming forward in time and seeing yourself as if you are at that place already.

Seeing what the payoff is, *right now*

What's so great about visiting your future self and envisioning how happy and healthy she is, how much she is enjoying life; is that you can see the payoff from changing how you eat rather than the short-term, *I can't eat unlimited chocolate anymore, boo hoo.*

The excitement for your goal will far outweigh your desire for fattening food. The future is brought closer to you and you can enjoy the benefits today while you are getting there.

Your *Thirty Slim Days* action tips:

Visit your future self and get ready to be inspired by *YOU*.

Choose a question from this chapter and start to find out **how awesome you already are**.

Ask what kinds of actions you think you might take as that **slimming success** in the future. Eat fresh organic produce? Be strict about three meals a day with no snacking? Have a daily yoga practice?

Whatever you list down, ask why you aren't doing those actions already? Can you **start one thing today**?

Day 17
Increase your self-care

Something I have realized about myself is that the more I slack off with my self-care, the sloppier my eating habits become. It seems that if I let one area go to the pack, everything else follows.

I love all the feminine girly parts of life, but I am also quite lazy, oops, I mean relaxed. If I was a millionaire I would pay people to do everything for me but, since I'm not, I do it myself. And when I talk about self-care, I mean to look after myself in all ways, not only the pretty, fun things.

All this to say, a big part of being a slender and happy person for me is to remember that self-care is not indulgent or something to feel guilty about: it's vital to my health, happiness and wellbeing. This in turn flows towards a happy home life, the love I have to give to others and how generous I feel towards the world in general.

Basically, caring for myself makes me a better person.

When I think of all the different kinds of self-care I *could* do that I would value and enjoy, the list is enticing:

Go for walks
Take yoga classes
Have my hair done
Look after my nails
Get plenty of sleep
Have time to rest during the day
Read novels
Read non-fiction
Create meals as if I am at a health resort
Journal
Meditate
Have a massage
Wash and blow-dry my hair
Apply light makeup daily

Most forms of self-care costs nothing

Looking at this list, there are only three items that cost money: going to a yoga class, having my hair done and having a massage. The rest are free. What sort of a twisted mindset did I have if I thought that self-care activities were self-indulgent?

I am naturally quite a thrifty person anyway, so I would only get my hair trimmed or coloured if I needed it. A massage once a month would be a big deal to me and my once-a-week yoga class also feels like I am quite spoiled.

Everything else needs me to give permission to enjoy myself and take a break. For some strange reason I find this quite difficult, so is it any wonder my subconscious has manufactured situations in the past where I relaxed and ate comforting foods to enjoy myself instead?

There are also other less tangible aspects of self-care that appeal too:

Being looked after if I am feeling fragile or tired
Feeling like I am good enough exactly as I am
Being grateful for my life instead of being an entitled brat
Giving love to myself as much as I love others
Not feeling like I have to be doing something every minute of the day
Feeling like I am making a difference
Not second guessing myself all the time
Not feeling guilty every day

Looking through these two lists, the overall feelings are laziness and guilt. Mmmm, what a pair of ugly sisters. And when I let them take over, chaos ensues. Laziness leads to slopping around, eating whatever I feel like regardless of the consequences, and guilt leads the way to rebellious eating. You may already know that rebellious eating does not involve fresh fruit or a colourful salad.

It is easy to see when I write it down that a way for me to eat better and be happy about it (maybe not even notice it) is to show these two negative emotions the door.

But how you can change how you think about your list of things that will make you feel good, when you can't be bothered doing any of them? Where do you get that kick-start from? Changing things a little bit at a time, that's how. Incremental upgrades lead to somewhere better. And sometimes just chucking guilt out the window.

Straightening out my priorities

An example is the yoga class I used to attend religiously years ago. Sometimes I attended once a week and sometimes twice. I loved going twice a week but the classes were expensive. I would often feel bad for spending that money; nothing to do with my husband saying anything, it was all in my head. Then, one day I let my concession ticket run out and didn't go again.

The crazy thing is, at that time I was still spending money on junk and snack foods. So... I was putting those ahead of a class that I enjoyed and had been getting excellent health benefits from. Great choice, Fiona.

I let my inner brat decide instead of making an intentional decision based on my values. At the time I thought, *Yoga classes are expensive, I'll give it a break for a while... Ooh, those chocolate almonds look good.* It took me a while to return, years actually, but I am pleased to be back at my yoga class and I spend the money I would have spent on junk food to pay for it. It might not be as much fun to my inner two-year-old, but the grown-up is in charge now.

Wrapping yourself up in a mini-retreat

Another form of self-care I love, yet I still have to push aside laziness every so often to do it, is having spa time at home – a mini retreat of sorts.

A mini spa retreat almost feels like a sick day from work to me, except that you're not sick, just tender of spirit. All obligations such as housework are put aside for a period, apart from light straightening up so that you can enjoy being in a tidy space.

I've never been on one of those expensive spa retreats (or even a cheap one) where you live at a five-star resort for a week or more and do yoga in the morning, have tropical fruit for breakfast and be pampered with massage and facial treatments. I have often fantasized about doing so, however.

What I love to do is recreate my own version at home. It is something to cocoon and cosset myself when I am feeling run down, burnt out or my mind needs some soothing. If necessary, I'll take a whole day or even a weekend, but mostly an evening is enough for me.

If you are feeling stressed out over weighing more than you'd like, having your own mini spa retreat is a beautiful way to comfort yourself when all you can think of is comforting yourself with food.

From the list of activities below, pick as many as you need to and wrap yourself up in them:

- Have a long shower
- Wash your hair
- Shave your legs and underarms
- Moisturize all over
- Apply light makeup or go bare-faced
- Blow-dry or straighten your hair or apply a serum and let it dry naturally in a loose bun
- Dress in clean, comfortable and attractive home loungewear
- Apply perfume
- Tidy up your bedroom and make the bed
- Find a book on your shelf you've been meaning to read – choose the one that appeals most
- Fill a big jug with water and place it on the coffee table with a glass
- Gather one or more cosy throw rugs – if it's summer, have them under you
- Bring a pillow down from your bedroom for the sofa

- Fill a foot-bath with warm water and whatever you have – Epsom salts, essential oils
- Place the foot-bath on a folded towel in front of the sofa
- Soak feet and smooth heels with a foot paddle if you have one
- Moisturize your feet with thick cream and put slipper-socks on
- Put one of your favourite feel-good movies on if you'd rather watch than read – the sillier and more light-hearted the movie the better

For food on your mini spa retreat, think what they would serve at the fancy places – fresh tropical fruit, herbal teas, lean protein, luscious salads. For some reason I imagine pomegranate seeds would be sprinkled all over the salad... Ask yourself what you would love to pamper yourself with that might be on the menu there.

Drink plenty of water throughout the day and if you feel weak and have cravings for your favoured unhealthy foods, lie down and take a nap.

If you don't have the house to yourself, let your family/house-mates know that you are feeling tired and plan to have a duvet-day.

The perfect end to your mini spa retreat day is to have a crazy-early night. I'm sure at the real spa weeks you are sent to bed as soon as it gets dark, and when I am feeling fragile this is exactly what I know I need.

Snuggle in with your book and know that tomorrow is another day. Repeat as necessary, or book in a regular evening once a week where you comfort yourself with some tender coddling.

The art of managing your mind

Some days though, even having a foot bath or blow-drying your hair is too much effort. On those days it feels good to simply go through your day asking 'What would I like to do next?' At first I thought when I asked myself that, the answer would be obvious – eat of course – but when I did, I found that was not the case.

What I wanted to do was all those sorts of things I had on my wish-list but never did, such as start a tiny craft project that I could complete in a day, reorganize my wardrobe or work on a writing project. When I put no pressure on myself, my excitement for these activities blossomed.

If, on the other hand, I had a free day with a short to-do list of:

Straighten wardrobe
Start writing project
Make patchwork cosmetic purse

I would rebel against my own well-meaning list and do none of it, choosing to go shopping for snack foods which I would then sit on the sofa all afternoon eating.

Looking at the big picture, it was easy to see that by letting myself enjoy life, do things that made me happy, rest every now and then and be taken care of sometimes; I would have much less of a need to comfort eat.

It's harder when you're in it, but it's not impossible. All it takes is a bit of faith that you do deserve to rest and enjoy your life, and not be a machine taking care of everyone else but yourself.

Your *Thirty Slim Days* action tips:

Are your **values** in alignment with how you spend your time? Some of my core values are:

Peace
Creativity
Simplicity
Health
Inspiration
Family

Ask yourself what you value, and then see if these values fit in with how you live your life.

List as many different types of **self-care** as you can, and see if you can do any of them more often. If guilt comes up, ask yourself truthfully if that emotion is founded on anything concrete, or if it's merely an old habit of yours.

If you had a **day to yourself** to spend exactly as you pleased, what would you do? Would you have an at-home spa day? Book in for a massage? Go for a walk and solo coffee with a book in the city? Take in a movie? Declutter your makeup?

Whatever it is you decide to do, do that. Choose something that won't take longer than a day if it is a project, and enjoy the satisfaction as you finish up. Make sure whatever you do on this day is because you want to do it, not because someone else said it was a good idea.

If all this seems like you are taking too much time for yourself and it would be selfish to, **start small**. For me it would be half-an-hour of reading time each day. Currently I book it in around 4.30pm and I look forward to it.

Have fun and remember, self-care is not an indulgence, it's a necessity.

Day 18

What would she do?

I woke up in the middle of the night and couldn't fall back to sleep because I was worrying about a trip to visit family that we were going on in a few days.

My worry was that I had put on some weight and had a sense of being out of control with my snacking. My more pressing worry was that none of my clothes fit nicely, particularly the few summer dresses I had, and where we were going was forecast to be warm.

I hated the idea of feeling bad about my higher weight and of my dresses hugging my 'curves'. I was getting myself so wound up and I knew I would never be able to fall back to sleep at this rate. Worries always seem worse at night, and I logically knew that, but I also knew that my concern was real – my clothes *were* tight and I *was* struggling to find clothes in my wardrobe that made me feel good. And my snacking *was* out of control!

As I lay there I used a technique designed to not only turn around your thinking so that you feel better, but that also gives you good, useful, inspiring information to act upon. I have used it before in various situations and it has never failed me. It goes like this...

You ask yourself 'What would a slim lady do in this situation? How would she live her life as a slim person?'

My mind immediately started flooding with positive ideas and statements and I knew that not only did I have to capture them because they felt so good and would motivate me in an effortless way, but also because I wouldn't be able to get back to sleep if I didn't empty them all out of my head.

I didn't want to switch my bedside lamp on, so I went into our ensuite bathroom and closed the door so I could turn the light on there and write them all down.

How would she live her life as a slim person?

She would eat for health and nutrition, not 'fun'
She wouldn't eat many sweet things
She would be organized with meals ahead of time
She would choose food based on the outcome she wants – feeling good, being healthy
She would know that a taste lasts only a short while, whereas being slim lasts all day, every day
She would feel empowered when choosing good nutrition over rubbish

She would know that it is completely up to her what she chooses to put in her mouth
She would know that cravings are not more powerful than she is
She knows she can be as slim as anyone else
She doesn't think about what to take away, she thinks what she could add to a meal
Instead of feeling ashamed of herself, she would feel empathy, optimism and empowerment
She would want to work out why she eats as does and support herself to find the answers in a gentle, non-threatening way.
She plans for her 'danger times' and looks for ways to switch things up to dislodge unhelpful habits
She has fun things to do that are not food-related
Rather than disliking junky snack foods, she chooses to be indifferent to them
She would be a selective and moderate eater
She would never give up

All of these statements came from inside my head, which means they are available to me and perhaps are my true self if only I listened. I can choose to be that person now and do all the things she does. I can behave as she does and choose to do as she does.

Brainstorming this list gave me hope that all was not lost, and it put me in a better frame of mind to deal with my clothing situation right now and eat better food to regain my slimmer self.

With my wardrobe, I had new motivation to sort through and create a mini-capsule to help me feel comfortable and attractive while I reset my eating and slimmed down my figure. It wasn't a very big collection of clothing I came up with, but I felt happy in it and the pressure came off.

Step away from your current situation and see *what could be*

Doing what I have done in the past only keeps me there. It keeps me in the same physical shape I am already in.

You might think, as I did, *But I am not that person, look at me, I'm out of shape, I eat junky food, I am out-of-control and I don't know how to stop.* I have had those same thoughts, and still can at times when I am feeling down.

But think about it this way – when you go on a trip somewhere, do you think about the place you've left, or the place you are going to? If you are planning to take a journey and leave home to drive to a city two hours away, are you constantly thinking of where you have come from? Thinking you'll never get there?

Or are you on the road, imagining what you are going to do when you arrive. You're not there yet, but you know you will be soon, and you know you're going to have a ball when you get to your destination.

It's the same with your physical shape. You know deep down that you could be slimmer and healthier if you really put your mind to it and that it *is* possible for you, but you keep coming back to, *But look how I am now, I can't change that much, I'll always struggle just a little bit, I might as well accept the way I am.*

I'm going to ask you to **forget** about what you look and feel like right now. Put your blinkers on and **only** focus on the new version of you. Imagine the woman you desire to be.

Step into her shoes, embody her

You might have a ritual when you do the grocery shopping each week of an Iced White Chocolate Mocha. You know it's a hip-widening habit but you feel deprived if you don't have one, yet you know ordering this drink doesn't align with the way you wish to be.

Ask yourself what *she* would do – your perfect future self. Would she have a sickly sweet creamy drink full of chemicals? Or would she savour a Café Crème or Americano. Ask yourself what she would choose, and have that. It changes the feeling from one of deprivation to empowerment (my ongoing theme and mantra).

I love the book *Jemima J* by Jane Green. The main character starts off overweight, watching the world go by but not participating in it because she is too busy eating for pleasure. A chance occurrence at her workplace, where a colleague photoshops Jemima's head onto a slender lady's body posing on a bicycle, inspires Jemima because she sees herself in a new way.

There is a scene in the book where the new Jemima, even though she hasn't lost the weight yet, visits a café and is inspired to order a sparkling mineral water rather than her usual order because she is choosing to step into the new version of her.

Call upon your chic mentors

Sometimes it is a helpful start to model yourself on people who inspire you too – your own chic mentors. In my life I have chic mentors that I know and are friends with; chic mentors that I don't know well but see around; and also well-known people whom I don't know at all, such as Aerin Lauder.

My chic mentors inspire me in different ways and give me ideas on living my most elegant life. I don't copy everything they do, but I borrow what is applicable to my own life and what appeals. I adapt details but use them in my own way.

I love to journal new inspiration to keep my ideas and thoughts fresh too, because after a while the newness can wear off. If I only have one page of notes to read over and over it quickly becomes stale. When I am creating new ways to inspire myself it means I am having fun with life and don't look for fun in other areas such as snack foods.

It's not all about chic and France and Europe either. I am also inspired by ladies from other European countries, as well as the United States; it's an endless list.

Here is my Californian girl inspiration that I came up with one day:

The Californian me – What would she do? How would she be?

She has a light and healthy tan
She has long hair with natural highlights
She wears cut-off jean shorts
She listens to Sheryl Crowe music
She laughs a lot
She eats salads
She drinks water from a big bottle
She has a sunny personality
She does yoga
She walks along the beach
She goes on hikes
She wears slinky leggings and little tops at home
She wears tunic caftan-style tops
She goes to the gym
She has a big, colourful salad for lunch
She keeps her apartment clutter-free and it is
    decorated in light and airy beach tones

To me, it doesn't matter that this might be an unrealistic magazine-version of what I think a woman who lives the beachy actress lifestyle might be like. I can freely borrow from television programs and movies because the result is a vision that inspires me – it doesn't need to be real. What is reality anyway?

Everything we see is filtered through our own unique lens, so why not change our sunglasses and look at life in a new way? That's what is excellent about coming up with your own inspiration – it is custom-tailored to speak to *you*. To give *you* new ideas. To shake things up, in a good way.

I often find I am more inspired to make positive changes after watching a movie than forcing myself to make those same changes. Maybe that old saying relates to motivation as well – 'a spoonful of sugar helps the medicine go down'. By having an enticing new way of being to add a bit of pizazz to your life, you willingly make those positive changes that you could not be bothered to before.

After watching Monica Belucci in the James Bond movie *Spectre* I couldn't wait to write down my Italian inspiration:

The Italian me – What would she do? How would she be?

She makes no apologies for her curves
She wears glamorous eye makeup and has fun with her eyeliner techniques
She dresses with a little bit of flamboyance and sexiness
She flirts in a playful and natural way, with both men and women
She looks after her figure
She is adventurous with new fruits and vegetables

She takes time out to live a slow-paced European lifestyle

She takes care of her possessions

She listens to opera

She is sensual

She savours her coffee

She has exquisite skin and uses traditional products such as almond oil

She is not so serious

She is light in spirit and fun to be around

She focuses on good food and cooking rather than eating pre-made junk

She values her health and eats high-quality natural food

She touches people on the arm when talking with them

She is caring and maternal and wants to include others, draw them in.

She is warm and nurturing at the same time as being sexy

She is easy-going

She is good fun

She is a good conversationalist and joins in with thoughtful observations

She likes to cook for her family and she is very good at it

She is intelligent but doesn't try to dominate the conversation or show you how much she knows

She is comfortable in her skin

She is slim, but not skinny

She wears a lacy bra which you might get a peek of when she wears an oversize shirt

I love my Italian persona so much. Aside from the Parisian me, I think the Italian me is my next most influential. And in many ways Italian style is much more approachable and liveable. Still, I'm glad I don't have to choose one or the other, I can have both!

I hope you are not tired of my various ladies yet, because I have one more.

Another time when I was journaling, I had the vision of me in another reality: a parallel me. It wasn't like a visualization in that I wanted to live this woman's life, but she is me.

There is an old money area that I love to visit in the city where I live. The homes are stately and I imagine what it would be like if I lived there. Even driving through this area makes me feel good. People look after their homes, and their gardens are beautiful.

The Fiona who lives here is different to the Fiona who eats kettle corn for lunch and devours an entire large-size bar of sweet milk chocolate in the evening... I made some notes to capture this Fiona. Before I even wrote these down, I could act (and eat) differently. It felt gentle and enjoyable.

The other me – What would she do? How would she be?

My slim lifestyle inspiration. I am the Fiona who:

Lives in a spacious high-level apartment
Decorates in tones of cream
*Displays her needle point projects (in frames, as
     cushions etc.)*
Dines elegantly
Loves eating in moderation and feeling light
Walks to the local shops nearby
Has a clutter-free home that feels airy and light
Cooks with pleasure
Earns good money independently
Has a beautiful kitchen and streamlined pantry
Sips Lemon or Lime Perrier
Doesn't like anything sweet i.e. foods, perfume
Lights candles daily
Curates and edits her life on an ongoing basis
Wears size 'Small'
*Loves buying, preparing, serving and eating fresh
     food*
Cooks seasonally
Is focused on many different pleasures

As you can see, it is not only about food and eating, but about how this lady lives. Creating a whole picture brings her to life and allows me a glimpse of her world and shows me how I can create it for myself.

Surround yourself with inspiration

Upgrading your surroundings affects how you feel inside, so if you give your home a good clean and tidy, or even a single room or area; it helps you feel good which affects how you care for yourself.

Writing this inspiration made decluttering easier for me too. I simply thought to myself 'does Fiona have this in her spacious and elegant apartment?' and I had my answer straight away. It was a clear distinction and I could let go of items with ease.

Your *Thirty Slim Days* action tips:

Have some fun with this and ask yourself about your ideal self:

What would she do?
How would she feel about food?
How would she dress?
Would she have a relaxed relationship with eating?
What would her daily menu look like?
How would she behave when by herself?
How would she behave around others?
What kind of boundaries would she have?

There are **endless questions you can ask of this lady**; let ideas flow out of your head and onto paper (or screen). Don't filter or censor; simply write down everything you are given. Sometimes the most interesting information surfaces this way.

The best time to do this is either last thing at night or first thing in the morning, but I find any time of the day is good if you are inspired. If you watch a movie where one of the characters stirs you (even if he's a man; I was as moved by Daniel Craig's character in *Spectre*), make some notes detailing why they stimulate your creative mind.

Day 19
Have your portions be chic

My favourite way to make healthy ideas more palatable is to reframe them in an appealing way. We all know that one of the ways 'naturally' slim people stay slim is by eating smaller portions.

Think about the term 'portion control' though. It's not sexy is it? The word 'control' does not sound welcoming and fun. Or saying to myself 'just take a smaller portion' – well, that triggers the voice in my head which screams out, *It's not going to be enough, I'll get hungry.*

How about saying 'French-girl portion size', 'ladylike portion' or 'a dainty portion' instead? Much nicer. Next time you are serving up a meal for yourself or dithering over which size to choose in a café or restaurant, just think, 'I am choosing the chic portion size; which size would *that* be?'

I hereby announce that I now eat 'chic' or 'dainty' portions. How much nicer does a chic portion size sound? And more attractive?

The chance to benchmark your portion sizes

I love to observe slim people eating when I am out, discreetly of course. Buffets are excellent for this. Whether they are dining with you or are strangers at the next table, I love to see how much slim ladies put on their plate. Sometimes I am surprised at how small the portions seem and I realize how large mine have become.

My husband likes big portions (which he burns off by going to the gym) which makes mine seem smaller by comparison. On one occasion, I was shocked to see that my own 'smaller' portion was bigger than my dad's when we had him around for dinner and all served our own food. That definitely gave me a wakeup call.

It's tempting to pile everything onto my plate at a buffet or serve-yourself family dinner, but it's just as easy to take a tiny amount of the dishes I fancy, and get more later if I want. Usually I find I don't need to go back for seconds.

I don't snack between meals any more, but when I was still working up to that, I downsized my afternoon snacks by having chic portions.

I used to love my afternoon wind-down time for an hour or so before dinner with a book or magazine, a cool drink and something to nibble on. But I often (okay, always) took the nibbles too far and found it hard to be enthused about dinner. A solution that proved successful was to serve myself a helping and put the bag or container away – sealed up and stored.

Serving a ladylike portion in a pretty blue-and-white Spode bowl (it's like a sugar bowl or tiny cereal bowl size) and then putting the rest in the pantry meant I had a small portion and that was all. Sometimes I had to resist going back for more; and sometimes it was easy, I ate my portion and that was that.

I know potato chips aren't chic in themselves, but I do love them. I felt vindicated when I saw a photo spread of Aerin Lauder at home where one picture showed a small blue-and-white bowl of potato chips for a casual guest snack (where do you think I borrowed the idea for my Spode bowl from?)

Aerin is very slim, so I think she must practice portion control too. Or maybe, do you think that tiny bowl might have been for everyone and not just her? Oops.

I have seen many examples of 'portion creep' where breakfast dishes from yesteryear are compared with their modern-day equivalent; and how tiny a small portion of French fries or a small cup of soft drink was compared with what is considered small today.

What to do about portion sizes when you eat out

It can be hard to cut back portions though, with large-size servings commonplace. I often find that my eyes are bigger than my stomach, and when I am less than half-way through a meal I am full. Yet I doggedly carry on, eventually finishing my plate.

From a young age I have been trained to clean my plate, and I still do it to this day. I cannot abide wasting food, so I eat it all instead (which is wasting it in a different way, I know).

I am trying to train myself to leave a little bit of food on my plate but it isn't easy. It's fine to finish my plate at home, because I can give myself a smaller portion to start with. When my mind says 'that doesn't look like much', I tell myself that I can go back for more if I want.

But in restaurants where portions are huge, what can you do?

There are two strategies that I use depending on the situation. If it's an ethnic restaurant where it is commonplace to take 'doggy bags' home, I will eat half of my meal and ask for the other half to be put into a container. I plan this from the start of the meal, and half is always a perfect 'just enough' chic portion size. I then enjoy an Indian curry or Italian pasta dish for lunch the next day.

If we are at a fine dining restaurant or a place where it is not appropriate to take away from, I choose what I am going to eat. Always the meat or fish, then the green vegetables, then the starchy vegetables. It hurts me to leave protein or green vegetables behind, but I don't care so much for the potatoes or rice so I tend to leave most of those.

I have trained myself into this even though starchy carbohydrates used to be one of my favourite components of a meal. Once I learned how bad they are for your insulin levels I was put off them. Don't get me wrong, I still wish this wasn't the case, but I accept it and choose to keep rice, pasta and potatoes out of my diet as much as possible.

I make pasta or rice meals at home, but they are the exception rather than the rule. And potatoes are a once or twice a week thing rather than every day.

With portion sizes at home, it's easy. I simply cook less, or make a lunchtime ready-meal if there is a lot. I sometimes even do my Indian restaurant trick if I have served myself too much – I'll eat half, then scoop the rest into a Tupperware container for the next day's lunch.

Your personalized physical guideline

It can be tempting to keep on nibbling, but it feels far nicer an hour afterwards to have had a moderate portion. Did you know the physical rule that your stomach is the same size as your closed fist? I invite you to make a fist and take a look at it – it's quite small isn't it?

Your stomach can stretch; it's not fixed at that size, but do you really want that? Do you want to get used to bigger and bigger portions over time? It's quite horrible when you think about it, but it's what we are doing when we let our portion sizes get bigger and bigger incrementally.

Having daintier and more ladylike portions feels strange at first, but it won't be long before our stomach shrinks and we are happy with slightly less.

It takes three weeks to change a habit, so it will only be for a relatively short time that these changes cause discomfort when your mind wants you to go back for seconds or serve a bigger helping in the first place. After three weeks it will begin to feel more normal that your portions are smaller.

Imagine how pleasant it would be to eat a meal that comfortably sits in your stomach and is digested easily. Over time you will naturally desire smaller portions; this will lead to less food consumed overall and a slimmer physique.

Quite often I close my fist and look at it when serving up or deciding what size I want to order. It gives me an instant visual on what a good portion size for me is. This rule works well, because our fist is in proportion to our body size.

Remember, a man will likely have a bigger fist than a woman. Mother nature is very clever, she gives us all our own correct portion size. My husband's fist will be bigger than mine, and a child's fist is smaller.

One chic mentor experience I'd rather forget

I remember a group dinner I attended, which was served buffet-style. One of the ladies in attendance is a secret chic mentor of mine. I observe her because I am fascinated at how she always looks put together, yet relaxed; curvy yet slim.

I only see this friend once or twice a year, and I always look forward to seeing what she is wearing, her mannerisms and how she speaks etc. She really is a delight to be around.

I realize this might sound like I am some sort of a spy, and maybe I am; for chic reasons only though. What I observed at this particular dinner was the portion size she served herself.

When we are home, serving up our own meals, it can be easy to add a little bit more, then a little bit more, and over time our portion sizes creep up. We cannot benchmark ourselves with others except those we live with, and I live with a man who likes big meals.

At this group dinner I was given a reminder that indeed, my portion size creep was out of control. I admit, I had made some bad choices at the buffet table and dished up too much of one item; then, when I had added everything else there was to choose from, my plate was heaped high.

My chic mentor took the tiniest amount of everything. Honestly, her portions were *minuscule* – some servings of food were as small as a matchbox! And dessert was the same.

To my mind, her dinner and dessert plates looked like kiddie plates served up – and mine looked like a lumberjack was about to tuck in. My secret chic mentor is curvy, but slim, and I can see why. Portion size.

Buffet strategies

Having a think about this dinner, there are two ways to go with serving yourself at a buffet.

One. You can take a tiny spoonful of everything. This would be a great option if all the dishes look amazing and you can't choose.

Two. You can decide as you stand there about what you are going to have and what you are going to leave behind. Choose your favourites from what looks nicest, and don't worry about the rest.

And always, of course, choose to have the one serving; no going back for seconds.

Portion strategies at home

When I serve myself dinner at home, often I am full before I have eaten even half of what's on my plate. That's telling me something, right? Going back to the 'closed fist' stomach size explanation above – *that's* why. That's why I am full with only half of my dinner.

Something that I would consider looks like a kiddie-size meal is probably a good portion size for me to have. It's not that I am trying to be ridiculous and eat very little to be skinny; it's that my eye doesn't know a reasonable serving size anymore and I want to get back to having my stomach feel comfortable after eating.

That's why I don't mind resetting my meals with external help (such as a weight loss book or menu plan) every so often. I can get a good reminder on what a portion size looks like.

The trick to being satisfied with smaller portions is to lessen the carbs and up the protein. Carbohydrates don't keep us full for very long; they are instant energy and can be converted to fat on our body very easily. Protein on the other hand is slow-release energy that the body does not store well.

By eating a little more protein and a little less carbohydrate, you are setting yourself up for a number of hours of fullness – enough to get you through to your next meal. Plus, you are not storing fat.

What this means at dinnertime is that you would have one extra slice of roast chicken, and one less roast potato. Simply tweak the quantities. My husband and I enjoy roasts a lot; they are an easy meal to make and there is leftover cold meat for our lunchtime salads.

I used to have two pieces of potato and my husband would have three or even four. Since we started cutting back the carbs, we have replaced potatoes with other options.

Now, a typical roast meal might include roasted onion, carrot and pumpkin along with steamed green vegetables. Every so often we will share a potato and have a small half each, but mostly we don't, and we don't really miss it. In addition, I now have maybe three big slices of roast meat, whereas before I had less.

It is still a delicious meal and fills me up, but it feels lighter afterwards and is also going to have less impact on my insulin levels and therefore my weight.

Your *Thirty Slim Days* action tips:

Find a name for smaller portion sizes that sits well with you – whether it is chic, petite, dainty, French-girl, or elegant. Imagine how nice it will be to have '**elegant portion size**' be your mantra for serving up your own food or how much you choose to eat. Get into the habit of keeping your mantra in mind at mealtimes.

By the same token, get into the habit of checking in with **the size of your closed fist** to anchor your new serving sizes. When you are serving up your meal, look at the plate, look at your fist; then decide whether you are going to put more on your plate or not.

From now on, **look at your portions with detachment**. Ask yourself if you would be happy to serve that portion up to a slim and elegant girlfriend you were hosting. Have someone you know in mind; someone that you look up to as a selective and moderate eater. This one always works for me!

Day 20
Love and praise yourself

A huge part of my issue with food, eating and weight, was the constant criticism of myself. Growing up I always thought that being a perfectionist was a good thing; I mean, it sounds good, doesn't it? With the word *perfect* in it? Who wouldn't want that?

It wasn't until I was a grown-up that I discovered it was *not* a good thing to be a perfectionist. Now, I know that being a perfectionist is a deadly affliction that will keep me frozen in indecision and inaction, and is a sure way to cultivate low self-esteem.

I never wanted to be too big for my boots (being 'up yourself' is frowned upon in New Zealand), so I would rarely give myself praise. More often the internal dialogue was looking at everything I had done wrong, not completed and how lazy I had been lately. Self-deprecation was a common theme and I thought that making jokes about my shortcomings was a good way to be funny.

Thankfully I have learned a lot in my study of personal development over the past decades, and I think I can say I am at the stage now that I truly do feel happy in myself. I feel like I am enough. I do enough and I have enough. Not one-hundred percent of the time, but a lot more than I used to.

When I was younger I had the constant feeling that I was going to get into trouble; I hadn't done enough for other people in my life and that I needed to be perfect for people to like me. *If they knew the real me, they wouldn't like me at all.* It was exhausting.

If this sounds like you, can I share what has helped me?

Listen to your self-talk

The number one thing to do right now, is stop criticizing yourself. It's probably going to be difficult because you have been doing it for a long time. But stick with it, because you *can* change your thoughts and it *does* get easier.

Next time you catch yourself thinking, *Ugh, I'm so fat and stupid*, stop yourself. Rephrase it in a more loving way, like you would talk to a dear friend if she had made an honest mistake. When you think about it, would you speak to a friend the way you speak to yourself?

Listen in and when you say something in your mind that you don't like; know that it is an old habit. Change it to the opposite saying, repeat it to yourself a few times and let it sink in. You can't delete thoughts, but you can overlay them with nicer and more helpful thoughts.

I used to be awful to myself. When I started saying nicer words, it felt strange, but good. How do you start to say nice things to yourself without sounding silly though?

The best way I have found is to think about all the phrases that you'd love to hear from someone else, such as:

Hey, beautiful.
That outfit really suits you
I love you, you're perfect the way you are
You are the light of my life
You can do no wrong in my eyes
I have unconditional love for you
I love you so much
You mean more to me than anything
You did a great job today
You are a wonderful sister/mother/daughter/
  friend/wife

Why not say one of these to yourself? Did you know that praise from yourself means more than praise from others?

Next time you feel down because a colleague, your husband or sister did not notice your new hairstyle, weight loss or mention a job you are proud of; say it to yourself. Say it out loud if you are alone, and especially say it to yourself every time you happen to be in front of a mirror.

Get into the habit of praising and loving yourself and *it will change your life*. Don't worry, you won't become big-headed or insufferably obnoxious. All that will happen is that your life will get better; you will become nicer to those around you and you will also subconsciously inspire others with your actions.

Why we put ourselves down and what to do about it

When I think back, it was habitual for me to put myself down to make others feel okay: I'd tell myself off for mistakes that sometimes weren't even my fault and berate myself every day of the year for eating badly, not exercising that day, looking awful in my clothes... the list was endless. It didn't feel good yet I still did it, because it was a habit I never thought about.

I promise you, there is another option, and it is to treat yourself like a queen, a precious beauty, a pearl, a jewel; because you are all those treasures and more. It sounds like a total cliché I know, but it's true. You have a worth that is priceless, so embrace it.

If you still can't see it, consider your loved ones. Do you think of them that way? I'm sure you love them to pieces (most of the time). So why not yourself? The best thing too, is that you can *become* that jewel by treating yourself as one. How beautiful is that?

Accepting and loving yourself has only good consequences

What about your body though? Are you afraid that if you accept and appreciate your body exactly as it is today, that you will get bigger and bigger? That you will eat and eat unchecked until you pop?

It won't happen. The act of accepting, loving and forgiving yourself will do the exact opposite. It will bring peace and calm into your mind and allow you to take healthier actions more effortlessly; because if you really loved yourself, you'd want the best for yourself.

The quickest way to see a point objectively is to take it back to someone else; if you loved someone so much and genuinely cared for their happiness and wellbeing, would you punish them by forcing them to eat unhealthy food and snack all day so that they felt sick, fat and unmotivated?

It doesn't sound very nice, does it, and I'm sure you wouldn't do that, just as I wouldn't. But... we have done it to ourselves; I have anyway. Many, many times. How nutty does it sound when you spell it out like that? Pretty nutty, I tell you.

This approach clearly doesn't work (I've proven that, and you may have too), so let's try the loving approach, like a kind mother would take. If you were the kind mother to yourself, you would coax yourself along and lovingly steer yourself in the right direction. You would want you to eat foods that nourish and support your health and wellbeing.

You would want you to be healthy and happy. You would tell you that you are enough, exactly as you are. You would hug you and fall to sleep at night letting you know how loved you are. You would love you unconditionally, even if you had made a mistake.

Maybe you grew up without good role models for body confidence, so all this loving talk feels quite ridiculous to you. Maybe the females in your life were constantly on diets, and talking about being fat when they weren't. Maybe they were critical towards *your* looks.

All of us have things we don't like about ourselves and features that we are self-conscious of. When I was pondering this blatant self-criticism that so many of us have, a vision popped into my mind of another way to be.

Create a compelling alternative vision for yourself

In my vision I was a tourist in Paris. I was strolling the streets with my love when we entered a boutique. I saw that the proprietor was a lady my age or a bit older. She was elegant, chic, stylish and very French-looking, but she didn't look young or perfect.

She had wrinkles, puffy eyes and other imperfections, but I imagined her with distinctive makeup and a hairstyle that suited her and her personal style; she was dressed with aplomb.

This image popped into my head that I could be that lady, that distinctive lady who owned her age, did not worry about her face slowly melting over the years, and simply enjoyed life and embraced her elegant femininity.

Where did we get it from that to be attractive and lovable also meant that we had to be perfect? It actually makes me sick that this is so ingrained in us and it has made me change my thinking, and decide not ever to complain about my looks or my age.

Will you join me in vowing not to denigrate your appearance? I think this will help with self-criticism and learning to be nicer to ourselves. In the past I couldn't even walk down the hall into my office without looking at my legs in the dress mirror at the end of the hall and automatically thinking, *Look how fat my thighs look.* It was automatic! There surely must be more positive and productive thoughts to think than immediately zero in on my thighs.

This is where emotional eating comes into it. We eat something comforting to make ourselves feel better, but it's only because we've been mean to ourselves in the first place that we want it, and our self-criticism was about being overweight! Something has to stop this unpleasant circle and I think it all starts with loving ourselves unconditionally.

My house and my car are not fancy at all, although both are perfectly functional and attractive in their own basic way. One day I hope that we can have a nicer home and a newer car, but do you think I wait until that day to show love and care to my home and car?

No! I appreciate and take loving care of both of these possessions *as if* they were my dream home and a newer car. What better way to practice? I can easily see that by looking after what I have now, I am not blocking myself from having fancier versions in the future. Quite the contrary – I am bringing them closer to me by treating my current home and car like they are my dream-come-true.

It's exactly the same with our physical being. By treating ourselves as if we are already that slim, healthy, vibrant and beautifully alive woman now, we are bringing her into our existence one day at a time.

We can dream of our future body where we are slimmer and healthier and our clothes look amazing, yet we can also enjoy our body right now. We can nourish her and be nice to her, clothe and groom her.

It feels much better to love yourself exactly as you are, rather than fighting with the image in the mirror. Have compassion for yourself and treat yourself as if you were your favourite and most loved person in the world.

Giving love to yourself in other ways

Some of us confuse food with love. Thinking back to my childhood again, I have memories of the treat and junk foods that were my downfall as a grown-up being entwined with love.

My nana buying us pick'n'mix chocolates from Woolworths on a Friday evening for the weekend. Being given a Cadbury Easter egg with chocolate buttons at Easter time. These were given with love by people who loved me and whom I loved back.

As an adult, I gave myself love by eating as much chocolate as I wanted to. And why did I do that? Because I was still so critical and perfectionist towards myself that I needed some loving. My inner talk was negative about my body; it was controlling about what I ate, and I rebelled.

Then, I gave myself love with sweet treats which meant I gained weight and only made my dictator voice worse. It's a vicious circle and I think it is heartbreakingly common, but that doesn't make it any easier to live with.

Again, you need to break the circle. If you show yourself love and compassion and treat yourself well, you won't need to gorge on treat foods to feel loved. You won't need the comforting taste of chocolate in your mouth as much.

I find it helpful remembering this link, even today. Seeing it in black and white shows me how absurd it is

– like a connection a child would make! And... I was a child when the connection was established.

It feels so good to let all that angst go, surrender to what is and love myself exactly as I am today, while also looking forward to improving my health one day and one meal at a time.

To support this positive frame of mind, I asked myself:

How can I give love to my body?

Focus on good health
Keep in mind a positive outcome
Think how easy it is for me to be slim and healthy
Enjoy feeling light with nutritious foods
Sleep well
Keep hydrated
Speak positively to myself
Give love to health
Look at all the things that go right for me
Imagine it's a year from now and any current issues
      are long-forgotten
Be open to my darling's support
Treat myself with compassion
Appreciate my good health
Rest sometimes
Be organized to feel peaceful

I also asked 'What do I already love about my body?' Surely there must be good points, right? Once I started writing it wasn't hard to carry on, and the list made me feel much better about myself:

What do I already love about my body?

My height – 5 foot 7
My shoe size - size 38
My slender fingers
My nice fingernails
I am in perfect health
My eye colour – grey/blue/green
My fair colouring
My golden-beige hair colour
My soft, moisturized skin
My nice boobs
My round bottom
My nice ankles and wrists
Good eyebrows
Straight nose
Good cheekbones
Youthful face
Can walk for one-hour plus
Long legs
Feminine figure
Perfect eyesight

This list didn't take me long, and I'm sure yours won't either. There will be features and attributes you like (or even love?) about yourself, and if you get stuck, think about compliments you have received from others. Write those down too.

Read this list when you start feeling picky and critical of yourself to help shift yourself to a better frame of mind. Feel gratitude for your fabulousness.

Your *Thirty Slim Days* action tips:

Do you think you have room for improvement when it comes to self-love? If so, make the decision to **stop being mean to yourself**, from *today*. Notice the thoughts as they come, and quickly replace them with something nicer. Keep a mantra in mind so that you don't have to think too hard.

I love to say to myself 'I am enough', borrowed from UK weight loss hypnotherapist Marisa Peer.

I am enough
I have enough
I do enough

There is a great YouTube video of Marisa Peer which I love to re-watch every so often. She speaks such good sense, and she's funny too. You can find it here: https://youtu.be/lw3NyUMLh7Y If you cannot use the link, search on YouTube for 'I'm not enough Marisa Peer'.

Think back to childhood and ask yourself whether habits and beliefs you picked up then, you still carry with you now. Are they serving you? If not, **give those beliefs back** to the person you received them from. You don't need to talk to that person; you can do it by yourself.

You might have conversations with yourself like this:

'I know my mum loved me by giving me a welcoming snack after school on a rainy and cold winter's day and I loved my hot Milo and toast with butter back then, but I am a grown-up now. I can show love to myself without feeding myself food that isn't necessary and will make me put on weight. I now choose to show love to myself with fresh healthy food and nurture myself in other ways.'

'When I was growing up, I heard that as a female you will continue to put on weight each year, and that it is unavoidable because your metabolism slows down. Proof of this was shown in the roundy figures of my older relatives. Now I know better. There is plenty of evidence all around me that show you can get better as you get older. I see ladies of retirement age who are slim and attractive and living vibrant and happy lives while dressing in a youthful and stylish way. That is me!'

Note down:
All the compliments you'd love to hear from others
How you can give love to your body
What you already love about your body, exactly as it is now

Read these lists for reassurance when you are feeling critical of yourself or like nothing is going right. They will comfort you.

Day 21
Be the queen of your life

What does being queen of your life have to do with being slim and gorgeous? Well, I'm so glad you asked. Can you imagine a queen, whether a real one or a fairy-tale version, moping around eating herself through an emotional calamity? No, me neither.

The queen in my mind would have high standards. If something was bothering her she would identify what it was and fix it. She would not stuff her feelings down with food.

Seeing yourself as a queen can enhance your life and make your journey to greatness (and slimness) easier and more enjoyable. In addition, you will gain other benefits outside of your focus area of health and losing weight.

A queen has many and varied qualities. She is elegant and feminine but strong and practical too. A queen gets her work finished and does what she needs to do. She knows that being queenly is not a temporary thing that she is going to try for a while. Being this way is her life's calling, her duty. By forgetting that she is letting herself down.

Think about Queen Elizabeth II. She has reigned as the Queen of England for sixty-five years. From the documentaries I have viewed, she treats her queendom as her job for life. She looks genuinely happy about it too. She doesn't complain that she can never retire from it and she does her job to the best of her ability every day.

It is the same for us. We can choose to be queen from today onwards. We can choose to be our best and most regal self, doing what needs to be done at the same time as enjoying our life.

The queen has work to do almost every day of the year, even at her age of ninety; truthfully, I don't know if I would want her job.

But look at the life she has led. It is hardly austere. She hasn't been living in a shack being the martyred queen. No, she enjoys her surroundings – the castle with the huge grounds in the centre of London; her holiday palaces; the royal ships, trains etc.

We might not have those resources; I personally don't own a palace, but it shows me that we don't need to sacrifice ourselves as is so common for women to do. We can choose to surround ourselves with our own brand and level of luxury and enjoy our life without guilt.

How does this translate to being slim though?

A queen chooses never to lower herself by consuming rubbishy snack foods. It is not queenly to eat cheap junk food to satisfy cravings. She chooses to eat high quality foods and nourish herself exquisitely.

She also chooses to **value herself like a queen** and knows that she requires rest in order to present her best self every day. A queen is not being selfish when she decides that she is going to have an early night with a book and a cup of tea because she has had quite a few banquets to attend this week.

She does not feel like she is depriving her family if she takes a solo stroll around the estate with her corgis to **tune into her thoughts**, or around the neighbourhood as I do. She knows that she needs her daily walk to feel and look her best and she doesn't feel pressured to skip her alone time on the days when there is a lot to do.

A queen sets up **routines which support her**. She rises at the same time each morning and retires to bed at a reasonable hour. She takes care of what she has to during the day so that she doesn't find herself finishing off jobs late at night.

A queen has boundaries. She isn't at the whim of others who use her to make their lives easier. She is kind and benevolent but also unyielding. A queen knows that if she gives in to others demands all the time it will erode her standing. She knows that people respect her when she sets and keeps boundaries.

By being this way she has no need to eat to comfort herself because she has not had a moment to herself all day. **She views food in its proper place** – as enjoyable fuel to partake in three times a day. She is not obsessed with what yummy thing she is going to eat next; no, she is focused on the task at hand and knows that her next meal will come soon enough.

A queen is practical. She doesn't sit in her palace being helpless and with no clue. If she lost her castle and all her money tomorrow she would still be okay. She knows how to feed herself. There are certainly skills she might have to learn, but she is intelligent and focused and knows she could easily do that.

A queen practises superb self-care. If the funds are available, she has a monthly massage and loves every minute of it. She attends yoga class that makes her feel so good afterwards. She chooses the high-quality chocolate or beautiful flowers when grocery shopping.

If a queen finds herself in times of austerity, she adjusts accordingly but **never drops her standards**. She knows that daily walks are free, and that reading uplifting material will help keep her in a positive state of mind.

She knows that it is only temporary and that there are so many no-cost activities she can still do. She might have cancelled her massage appointments, so she chooses to massage her own feet with a moisturizing cream instead. It feels blissful before she hops into bed. She also applies a face mask once a week during her at home spa time.

A queen balances family and public life. She is pleasant to those in the public sphere; perhaps colleagues or people she comes into contact with during her daily rounds, but she doesn't let them rock her. She avoids unpleasantness wherever possible and does not get involved in disputes between others. She keeps her eyes on her own path and lives a beautiful life to the best of her ability whilst also being of service to others.

Create your own list of queenly behaviours

For me, keeping the queen archetype in mind helps me be slim in many ways.

I stop being a brat about the food I want to eat and instead choose foods that befit my queenly role

I overcome and rise above pettiness which can lead to comfort eating

I find the strength to carry on with my healthy plans when it would be comfortable to go back to the way I ate before

I do what it takes to succeed in my vision of a healthy and slim life

I take the long-term view (being my ideal weight) rather than the short-term view (how something tastes)

I have good posture that instantly makes me appear slimmer and is better for my breathing and overall health – a queen stands as straight as Grace Kelly

I decide how I want to be and I follow through with that

I am decisive rather than wishy-washy

I set boundaries for myself and others and I uphold them

I have dignity – this transcends dashing to the supermarket because I have a craving

I have high standards in not only what I eat, but in every area of my life – what I wear, how I live, how I behave, and the people I associate with

I continue to uplevel my environment in small increments – my fridge and pantry are clean and filled with life-enhancing foods; my closet is organized and attractive with clothes that fit me and reflect my personal style well

I have firm boundaries at the same time as being kind and caring

I have a crystal-clear vision of how a queen lives and acts to guide me

I accept help from others and expect them to fulfil their roles as well

I can become the queen of my life by adopting these guidelines, and I do them in the first place because I am thinking of myself as if I am a queen already. I am willing to think of myself as queen and become that person I imagine.

I know that I will have times when I fail, but I also know it will not mean that I am a failure – because I carry on. I can only be a failure if I quit. I grow stronger because I move past issues big and small and continue with my quest. I don't let one day of bad choices be the end of my slim dreams. I pick up and carry on from the very next meal.

Do you think a queen never makes mistakes? That she never overeats in response to an internal trigger? I'm sure she has done. The difference between the women who make it and the ones who go back to how they were; is that queens get back on their horse straight away.

Everyone is allowed a blip; no-one is perfect. I don't let a mistake dictate that I am not meant to be a queenly success. I take it as part of being human and continue resolutely on.

You grow stronger in doing so, because strength is formed when you move past failure. You will then feel just as happy, probably happier than you were before. You rise again like the queen you are and take everything in your stride.

The alternative is for you to play it so safe that you will never make mistakes. This is not what human beings are designed for though. If we are not willing to do new things we will become stagnant. It pays to be bold, because we are all meant for a level of greatness which can only come to us once we take the next step.

You are a queen; own your greatness and be fabulously and successfully slim in the process.

Your *Thirty Slim Days* action tips:

Have a small symbol of your queendom to remind you often of your regalness. In the beginning it is helpful to have reminders. Once you have practiced this for a while it becomes automatic. A small crown on your keyring, a lipstick in a gold case, your signature perfume, even looking upon yourself as a queenly being. Queen Fiona has quite the ring to it, I think. How does your name sound?

Have a mantra that suits you. I love 'I am the queen of my life'; or I talk to myself as Queen Fiona, if I find myself being slovenly and entertaining thoughts of terrible food. This elevates my behaviour in a second.

Ask yourself what your queenly vision is. Do you see yourself as that regal lady? List out all the ways you would love to be the queen of your life then start living that way. There is no time like the present. You don't need to be all bossy about it; simply begin *acting is if*.

Day 22
My love-hate relationship with sugar

The simple fact is that sugar is everywhere we turn. Over the generations, it has changed from a rare treat to something that many of us consume in large quantities. We know how bad sugar is for our health, yet we eat more than ever.

I've seen shocking statistics at just how much sugar Westerners eat and the scary thing is, it's becoming normalized for younger generations. Instead of the 'old-fashioned' meat and three veg being an everyday meal, adults and children alike are now opting for a fast food meal as their norm; comprising a burger on a sugar bun (sugar is added to hamburger buns for taste and longer freshness), sugary mayo and sauces, starchy fries, a sweet drink and sugary soft-serve ice-cream with sugar syrup on top.

Sugar is being added to many different food ingredients and it seems that there is becoming a real divide between the organic, gluten-free, paleo crowd and those who subsist entirely on processed food.

Even though I knew logically I felt better and that it was healthier for me to eat simple, real, fresh, seasonal food that I've cooked myself; I still heard the siren call of salty, sweet, fried, processed foods that are manufactured and marketed to be addictive to our primal brains.

How did we end up like this?

The Western population has never been unhealthier than it is now. We have millions who are overweight, yet malnourished at the same time. How can that be, you ask? The human body, which has been perfected by nature over thousands of years, has a method to gain the nutrients it needs. You eat food, the body takes in nutrients; once the body has enough nutrition for its current use, you feel satiated.

Enter processed food. Processed food has been refined beyond recognition and most nutrients have been entirely stripped away during manufacture. Vitamins and minerals are added to make them seem healthy; colouring is also used to make the food look more appealing.

Your body does not recognise these foodstuffs and, as there are no nutrients to absorb, you don't feel satiated. You continue eating looking for the point of satiation, but this never happens. You might feel uncomfortably full, *yet you keep on eating*. Am I right? I know it was like that for me.

My poor body, trying to extract nutrients from this Franken-food and failing miserably. That's how I ended up grumpy and short-tempered short term, and battling frumpiness and weight problems long term.

Sugar and other processed foods are designed to be addictive to the human body; those naughty manufacturers know this and exploit it for their multi-billion dollar profits. I've read books that show how fast food companies plan how they are going to make their foods more addictive.

I know this sounds bad but it's true. And if you have ever tried to give up your 'favourite' downfall (I say favourite in inverted commas because we all have our love/hate foods that we simultaneously want to stop eating and don't ever want to be without), you'll know that it is near impossible with willpower.

Even knowing sugar and processed foods are bad news can't help us give them up; I know, I've tried many times over. Sometimes I'd think to myself, *This is ridiculous, just stop eating sugar and you'll be okay.* Which would work for varying lengths of time, from a few hours to a few days, but very soon I'd be back looking for my fix.

I know that saying fix sounds like I'm talking about a drug, and I am. Sugar is widely known as being as addictive as class-a drugs and is also called 'white poison'.

I knew all this, so why was I still craving it?

Sugar tastes nice, and the sweetness is something we will go to any lengths for, instinctively. But fruit tastes sweet as well. If I ate a piece of fruit that made my stomach feel uncomfortable and then gave me a headache later on, I'd probably not eat that fruit again.

With candy, ice-cream and sweet chocolate; despite the weight gain, sugar hangovers and knowledge that I was eating myself into a sugar-related disease such as type-2 diabetes, I'd still go back for more.

Sometimes it would be a week or two if I really made myself feel unwell the last time, but mostly it was every day that I'd look for something sweet to brighten things up.

For more than thirty years – over two-thirds! – of my life I have had a 'sweet tooth'. This charming sounding name glosses over the stress and anxiety that sugar has caused me, as I simultaneously wanted not to eat it, yet could not imagine what life would be like without it.

Like many people I'm sure, I associated sugar with good times. Candy at Christmas, birthdays, holidays and weekends. Chocolate Easter eggs. Having a glass of Coke on a Friday night for a treat as a child. Birthday cake and ice-cream at parties.

There were so many ways in which sweet foods were a happy part of my life. I would always try to get as much as I could as a child, but my parents and other adults were there to put boundaries on when and how much sugar I could consume.

I remember my mother giving my sister and I a chocolate bar to share. Her ingenious method was for one of us to cut and one to choose. She used the same when one of us poured the Friday night glass of Coke and the other chose. Of course it was in your best interest to be as even as possible, otherwise you had the smaller portion.

Most days cycling home from school involved stopping to buy a bag of sweets. I'd eat them all before I arrived home, my mouth parched at the drawing effect of sugar. Guzzling a big glass of water on top of all that sugar left me feeling sick, but I still did the exact same thing the next day because those sugary treats were just so delicious.

Maybe I'd grow out of it...

When I left home to start my adult life around the age of twenty I thought I would magically leave those kiddie sugar habits behind. But I didn't. In my first job, my morning and afternoon tea breaks were spent popping to the store downstairs to buy a bag of candy or a chocolate bar to make my desk work more interesting.

When I was young I never had a weight problem, thanks to my tall and lanky dad; however in my twenties I found myself stacking on the weight and I started feeling very frumpy. Most of my clothes didn't fit and the ones that did looked awful.

I joined Weight Watchers for the first time in my mid-twenties and was thrilled when the weight started coming off. I quickly realized that my meals were already quite healthy and merely needed small adjustments; however, my Weight Watchers points did not leave any room for candy, so my sweet treats were severely curtailed.

I managed to keep this up for a number of months. The combined actions of my healthier diet and daily walks meant I rapidly lost the weight that made me feel and look below-par. Eventually though, I came to the point where I was sick of counting points and feeling restricted.

You can imagine what I did next – I had a great big satisfying blow-out of all the foods I'd been denying myself, and revelled in not having any limitations. Very soon I was back to the same weight.

This is where I have been since that first dieting period twenty years ago and when my love-hate relationship with sugar gained traction. It's so hard to both crave sugar and know that it's the reason for your unhappiness, but I didn't know what to do.

Willpower only worked for a short time and I always ended back up at the same weight. I tried accepting my body at that weight and not worrying about what I ate but that didn't work either. I tried putting myself off the foods I craved by renaming them with unattractive names and imagining revolting people eating them. Did not work.

Changing my mind about sweet foods

I knew the key was how I felt about sugar. I still had those good childhood feelings of happiness, festivity, celebration and joy going on around sugar; and junk food manufacturers add to that with their advertising.

I recalled all the memories and wrote them down. I forgave each memory individually, as well as those who taught me that sugar was a treat; they didn't know any better themselves. I forgave myself for eating unhealthily and putting stress on my organs. I forgave myself for treating my body badly.

Having such a ferocious sweet tooth was seriously undermining my peacefulness and I decided that's what I wanted, even if my weight stayed the same – I wanted to feel peaceful around food and eating.

I knew there was some deep subconscious programming that told me sugar was a treat and that it made my life better, even though logically I knew this was not true.

Sugar is in many foods, not only the obvious such as candy, chocolate and ice-cream. When I dug down further though, I found I didn't have a problem with all sugary foods, only some. And by problem, I took this to mean foods that I couldn't stop eating once I'd started;

foods that seemed to have a hold on me and that I craved out of nowhere.

I didn't have an issue with dark chocolate for example, but I did have massive sensitivity and the associated cravings to candy, milk- and white-chocolate, ice-cream and a few other starchy foods such as popcorn and potato chips.

These were the foods that I wanted to eliminate from my life, but how?

The cure for me

One day I was pondering this, and my wise inner Fiona said to me, *This is ridiculous. The answer is right in front of you. You are dithering over what to do when it's obvious. You clearly are highly susceptible to sugar, much as an addict might be to drugs. Does an addict have a little bit of their drug each day for a treat? No. Do they have it only on weekends? No. The only way an addict can get better is by complete abstinence.*

So I did, and I still am. To begin with I didn't have anything with sugar in it, not even dark chocolate, tomato sauce or dried fruit (I never stopped eating fresh fruit though). Then, after a few weeks I slowly reintroduced the safer foods back into my diet; foods that didn't set off cravings.

I think some of us have this sugar sensitivity that those who don't can't see the problem with. They are the people who can have an open bag of sweet treats sitting in front of them and they don't have to finish it. I would love to be that person, but truthfully maybe I never will be, and that's something I have to be okay with.

I couldn't let it rule my life.

For the first four days I had a terrible headache and I felt like only sugar would fix it. I felt tired and my skin was tender to the touch. I actually felt like I was getting the flu, but I knew I wasn't. On the fifth day the fog cleared and I felt fantastic. It's been a while now and I have never looked back. I simply don't need sugar anymore.

How it feels on the other side

Supermarket shopping holds no fear for me now. I can shop for what is on my list and not find myself walking down the candy aisle. In the early days I avoided that aisle though, because I didn't want to tempt myself. It wasn't where I wanted to hang around anymore. When I needed more dark chocolate, I went to that aisle and then got out of there as quickly as possible, like I was in a bad part of town!

These days I feel peaceful around food. It's a wonderful feeling. I feel like a normal person now which I thought I never would.

That might sound overly dramatic but I was so envious of those people who could take or leave sweets and never seemed to snack between meals. Of course they were always slim, and I truly felt second-class next to them in my clothes too-tight with my sugar cravings sitting just beneath the surface.

Many was the time when I left a friend's after lunch together and literally fell in the supermarket door to buy a bag of sweets to eat on the way home.

I know there will be other ladies out there like me, because I've spoken to some of them. One lady in her fifties confided in me that she would volunteer to go and fill the car up with gas, just so she could buy a chocolate bar there and eat it on the way home. For those of us with a seemingly insatiable craving this is a very reasonable thing to do!

Her family teased her for her sweet tooth, so this way she could enjoy her chocolate in peace and her family would never know. Yes, she was always miserable about her weight too.

These days I feel true peace around food and it's amazing. I don't linger on the products that used to be my nemesis. I don't fantasize about how it would be great if I could still eat them. I simply turn my head the other way and think about what healthy food I am going to prepare that day.

It truly comes down to a decision, but it also helps to be prepared. I made sure I had plenty of fresh fruit and vegetables at home and I ate a good amount of protein at every meal.

Apart from fruit, everything I eat is unsweetened. This really helps. If a food product has sugar or some other sweetener in the top three ingredients, I don't buy it. And I don't have artificial sweeteners either, because even though these have no calories, they still set up cravings with their sweetness.

As they say, I am sweet enough – and so are you.

Your *Thirty Slim Days* action tips:

If this chapter resonated with you, here are some tips on how I successfully left sugar behind and in doing so gained a beautiful peace of mind.

Once you get past sugar's grip, the outlook on the other side is amazing. You have to pass through a brief storm to get there, but oh it's worth it. I have no sugar cravings and I look forward to my meals in a normal-person way.

Be excited for this, because it really is life-changing if you'll let it be. You are not giving up anything because those sweet foods are a false friend. They will lure you in and promise you happiness, but they are the complete opposite. In a way they are like the poisoned apple being offered to Snow White.

I felt empowered, not deprived when I said no to sugar, whether it was me saying no to myself or 'no thank you' to someone else who offered me a treat.

Because I was *always* up for afternoon tea/treats/sweets/cakes in the past, I had to have little excuses because I didn't want to draw attention to my lifestyle changes while they were still new. I didn't want to have to explain them to people and have them question whether it was too extreme to not have anything sweet ever again. I wasn't thinking about 'ever again'; I was just getting through *today*.

My favourite one when meeting a friend for coffee, was 'oh no thanks, I had a late lunch'. If someone offered me home baking that they might be offended if I said a straight-out 'no', I'd say 'That looks beautiful, I'll try some soon', but then of course that time never comes and they've forgotten about you trying it.

For me, it wasn't worth it to potentially trigger sugar cravings because I wanted to seem polite.

'That's not my food'... when my eye caught a poster for the newest chocolate bar flavour or a super-duper special snack offer at the supermarket, I'd say to myself, *That's not my food*. I borrowed this from Bright Line Eating's Susan Peirce Thompson and I love it. It's a simple statement of fact.

Since I was young I have never eaten ham, pork or bacon; I just never liked it. Whenever I see something, say a frittata in a café; if it has ham pieces in it, I immediately see what else there is for me to order, because I don't eat ham.

It's the same with sugar, processed and snack foods now; I pass on them because they are not my food.

Reminding myself of the alternative. I know that if I give in to a passing craving I will be right back at square one. I remember the miserable feeling of being led around by my cravings and know that I don't want to give away my control anymore. This helps me stay strong; and with all the days that pass, the cravings get weaker. Now, a craving can come into my mind as a passing thought and I easily flick it away. 'I don't do that anymore' I remind myself.

Rest. A few times, when the cravings were particularly strong in the beginning and I felt like I would collapse with weakness if I didn't eat something sweet, I lay down on the sofa and took a nap instead. Looking at it logically, it is far better to let myself rest if I am feeling tired, instead of pumping myself up artificially with sugar energy.

Please note that I have yearly blood tests to check everything and I don't have any issues with blood sugar levels. This is something you will want to have checked out first before you address your sugar cravings, to ensure you don't have any medical conditions.

For me, it was my inner toddler throwing a tantrum because I wouldn't buy her a bag of sweets.

Get your sweetness in other ways. I love sweet-smelling fragrances, candles and body products. I have a salted caramel candle that smells like home baking when I have it lit in my office and it's *gorgeous* to my nose. For some, having sweet scents around may trigger a craving for something sweet to eat; for me, it replaces it nicely.

I have heard of chefs who aren't tempted to eat what they have been cooking all day, because they feel satiated from the aroma of the food after many hours. This is how I feel about my sweet scents.

Don't give up. If you are a sugarholic like I used to be, I hope you find this chapter encouraging and that it gives you hope.

Day 23

Create your own inspiration

Motivation can need constant topping up during your weight loss journey, because your goal isn't going to show up at the door, tooting, *Come on, hop in*! You have to go after it, and you need to put in the effort before you see the results. This can be hard to start with, when you feel like you are depriving yourself for seemingly no payoff.

Decide that you want to be consistently slim and healthy, then go after it. It helps to begin with a childlike wonder that anything is possible; that beautiful Christmas Eve or birthday feeling when you were a child. Remember the sensation of possibility, wonder, hope, magic and excitement; all wrapped up in a beautiful sparkliness.

Anything *is* possible. If you can dream about it, you have it within you to create it. If you have achieved it before, no matter how briefly, it means you can do it again and *permanently* this time.

It takes managing yourself to get there, but also managing yourself once you are there; you need to keep the motivation up and be happy that the way you have lost weight will now be part of your daily life forever.

There are so many methods that teach us how to lose weight, but not many that show how to maintain it. That's where I have fallen down in the past; I'd go back to all the foods that I stopped eating, but of course as soon as I did that, the weight depressingly started coming back on again.

I'd forget that what got me there would keep me there, instead only cutting out those foods temporarily. Logically this makes no sense; is it any wonder I yo-yoed with my weight?

It's a matter of not giving up on your inspiration, and continuing with the same changes that helped you to your goal. These days I know there are some food items (none of them healthy, I might add) that I simply cannot go easy on; so I have made the decision to exclude them from my life. They are simply not worth the problems they create.

I used to fight that, and feel miserable that I couldn't have my favourite foods. But they were only my favourite foods because I ate them often. The more you have of something, the more you want it; this equally applies to healthy and unhealthy foods. There is some discomfort when you stop giving yourself the unhealthy foods that you know are at the root of your problems, but it gets easier.

Changing my thoughts

I have also made a change in the way I think about my former favourite snack foods. I have mentioned this change before but it bears repeating because it is so powerful.

I no longer feel deprived that I am denying myself my favoured treat foods. I now feel empowered that I am choosing to refuse them; empowered that I am no longer letting those foods be stronger than I am.

I feel empowered that I am choosing health and life over a temporary taste.

I feel empowered that I am choosing to look and feel amazing in my wardrobe.

It is the other side of the coin, and it's so much shinier. I was only looking at all the things I'd have to give up (such as overly sweet ice-cream, cheap milk chocolate in jumbo-size bars and all manner of food colouring bound in sugar and gelatine).

What will I gain?

Flipping over this same coin, I can see everything I will gain instead:

Being someone who values their health
Feeling vibrant every day
Being proud of myself
Having tons of energy
Feeling happy with myself
Looking nice in my clothes
Not feeling self-conscious
Feeling in control of my destiny

How motivating is that list, right? That's why it is so vital to revisit your inspiration to remember why you started in the first place, and why you want to keep on going; whether it's to your goal weight or maintaining your weight.

How can I?

Another way to create your own inspiration is to ask yourself 'How can I?'

How can I be in the best shape ever?
How can I make it fun, easy and enjoyable to reach my goal?
How can I learn to love eating healthily?
How can I enjoy being disciplined?
How can I feel empowered?
How can I be slim and healthy with ease?
How can I make it easy for myself to be skinny?
How can I love dressing myself in the morning?

I love asking myself questions such as these when I am having some quiet time with a pretty notebook or at my laptop with a fresh Word document. I choose a question and start answering it for myself. I don't stop until I come up with twenty ideas.

I also have a tiny notebook in my handbag which goes everywhere with me. I have created motivational lists in doctors and dentists waiting rooms, waiting in the car to pick up my husband and even while serving customers in our retail store. They were having a look around as I wrote thoughtfully in a small notebook while keeping in eye contact with them if they needed it. They probably thought I was ordering stock or making notes about a customer request. I love using pockets of time like this.

When I brainstorm answers for a question, some are outlandish but I still write them down. I let everything pop out of my brain because it is there for a reason and often there are grains of usefulness or even a completely new direction to go in which I hadn't thought of before.

One of the answers I came up with to the question **'How can I be in the best shape ever?'**, I almost didn't write down because I thought 'No way am I doing that'. It was 'Train for a body-sculpting competition'. Once I moved past the momentary resistance I wrote it down. Initially I felt that if I did write it down, I would *have* to do it. Not so! What this point achieved was to open my eyes to creating some simple weight-bearing workouts that I could do at home. And I only wrote down body-sculpting because I was trying to get to twenty ideas; throwing everything down on paper that I could think of.

The first answers are easy to come up with, and often what you are already doing or have done in the past. It's not until you really start to struggle for ideas that the gold comes out.

Here is my full list:

How I could achieve being a healthy, sugar-free and peaceful eater and in the best shape ever?

1. Make a decision to be so
2. Go organic
3. Inspire myself by curating my wardrobe
4. Try hypnotherapy
5. Try acupuncture
6. Research positives to healthy eating
7. Get into fitness – body sculpting
8. Turn obsession with eating to something else, such as writing
9. Be vegan or vegetarian
10. Go sugar-, dairy-, wheat-free
11. Address addiction as a whole life thing
12. Go into food rehab/detox
13. Positive thinking/visualization/picture me on health magazine covers
14. Meditation/prayer

15. Play a hypnotherapy track every evening
16. Model myself on healthy eating mentors
17. Take an online health/mindset course
18. Read my healthy eating inspiration every day
19. Journal – write my future into reality
20. Eat paleo/whole foods
21. Make it fun and exciting, and preferable to eating junk
22. Forget about the scales and my body; just focus on eating well and feeling good today
23. Rewrite my top ten health goals every day
24. Get food therapy
25. Hire a food/addiction coach
26. Gather a Pinterest board of fit and healthy slimming recipes
27. Try Emotional Freedom Technique

As you can see, some of these ideas are quite extreme. I won't act on all of them, but it shook my brain to see what would fall out! At this stage I already had the seeds in there that being addicted to certain foods could be one of my issues to address.

The next question stopped me focusing on all the ways I was out of shape and unhealthy, and instead looked at how I was already doing well. Doing this got me out of panic mode so I could feel relaxed; and when I feel relaxed I make better decisions. It feels good to be calmer when I am overthinking things.

How am I already slim and healthy?

1. I walk regularly around our neighbourhood
2. I eat fresh fruit and raw nuts for breakfast most days
3. I eat salad and protein for lunch most days
4. My treat lunch is fresh salmon and avocado sushi
5. My after-work drink is sparkling water
6. We cook at home most nights, mostly low-carb, high protein with good fats
7. I drink water and green or herbal tea, with not too much coffee or black tea
8. I go to bed early and I love it
9. I wake up at 6am most mornings
10. I eat multiple quantities of fresh vegetables each day
11. I keep my dairy intake quite low because it feels better to me
12. I no longer drink
13. I no longer eat sugar
14. I have learned to love savoury foods instead of sweet
15. I have learned to keep myself calm
16. I have created a low-stress life for myself
17. I breathe fully more often and no longer hold my breath as much
18. I eat three times a day and I don't snack between meals
19. I have trained myself out of a potato chip routine before dinner

20. Our home is stocked with good foods and no snack foods

The great thing about this inspiration list is that it could apply to when I was slim, as well as when I still had some weight to lose. There is nothing in it that says 'I am X weight'. It ended up being a set of guidelines that I could refer back to when I was feeling unmotivated.

Imagine if you asked yourself for forty or fifty ideas to a question, or even one-hundred? What sort of goodness could you come up with then?

I also love to brainstorm the questions to start with; they are as illuminating as the answers themselves I find. Here are some more of mine:

How can I be effortlessly slim my entire life?
How can I be healthy and have lots of energy?
How can I best look after myself?
How can I love foods that are good for me and dislike unhealthy and junk foods?
Can I really be overjoyed with my body?
Could I really learn to love physical activity?
Is it possible or do I even want to eat 100% natural and healthy, nothing processed?
How can I improve my health today?
How can I set our home up to be the easiest environment for good health?
How can I use my wardrobe as slimming inspiration?

Actually, that last question is so exciting to me right now, because I have been reading personal style books and re-organizing my wardrobe lately. Here is my list that I have brainstormed while writing this chapter.

How can I use my wardrobe as slimming inspiration?

1. Look to my favourite motivating movies i.e. slim NYC girls getting ready for their day at the beginning of *The Devil Wears Prada* movie.
2. Review my personal style files of stylish outfits, slim ladies and French Chic magazine articles.
3. Declutter items that do not make me feel elegant and sensual.
4. Twice a year – spring and autumn – do a complete wardrobe go-thru and remember my vision of a bijou Parisian boutique to keep my focus. Look at my closet as my own personal Paris boutique and treat it accordingly.
5. Work on refining my personal style – look for inspiration to my style icons such as Coco Chanel.
6. Create a series of uniforms that I adore for summer and winter dressing.
7. Be ruthless and unapologetic about getting rid of items that are not perfect for the image I wish to portray.
8. Include what I wear at home in this mindset as well – underwear, nightwear, lounge-wear.

9. Look into a sewing course to get back into making my own clothes – fashion design for myself and creating perfect pieces.

10. Bring the essence of Paris into my daily dress – think Audrey Tautou's insouciance; the simplicity of Ines de la Fressange.

11. Have fewer possessions of higher quality. Over time weed out those items that do not fit this vision.

12. Look at my exercise clothing and replace items that are shabby – they don't have to be expensive.

13. Enjoy creating a capsule clothing collection for the season that has a cohesive colour scheme which looks expensive and luxe – camel, oatmeal, black, navy, red, stripes.

14. Choose high-quality clothing items by considering the purchase and making the best choice at the time when I need to replace something.

15. Make it a delight to get dressed in the morning because everything hanging or folded in my wardrobe I love, fits me well and portrays my personal style and the woman I want to be.

16. Style my closet so that when I open the doors at any time of the day I am thrilled with what I see.

17. Declutter and organize my closet so that there is plenty of space, shoes included; nothing is messy and I can see everything at once.

18. Have at least one special occasion item that I can't wait to wear; that way I won't freeze in horror at a formal invitation.

19. Curate my wardrobe so it gives others an instant and consistent idea of who I am. Choose clothing which accurately reflects me, yet sometimes surprises others with little twists that I like to include to keep things fresh.
20. Dress in the simplest way I can since I feel best in outfits that are simple but luxurious with an accent accessory. Choose tailored and fitting clothing that flatters my figure and helps me feel pulled together.

Exciting ideas will appear as if by magic

Now the interesting thing is that some of these answers really surprised me. I don't consider myself to be *that* fashiony. I like to keep life simple and I don't really read fashion magazines. I like to be able to put my outfit on in the morning and forget about it.

But some of the answers I came up with tell another story. They say I am inspired by an elegant and considered wardrobe. That I am inspired by the mythical ideal Paris girl. Over the years I thought I had grown away from her and towards a simpler and 'me' way of dressing, but she is obviously still there. She's tapping me on the shoulder, saying 'don't forget about the sparks of inspiration that keep things exciting so that you won't turn to food for that instead'. How fascinating.

This is the kind of inspiration you can create for yourself that is custom-blended for your taste. And who wouldn't want a bespoke experience like that?

Your *Thirty Slim Days* action tips:

Create your list of questions – why not aim for one-hundred questions? I did this once; it was across all areas of my life, not just slimming and health. I still read through that list (and my answers) today and find myself re-inspired by it. Write down your top one-hundred questions that you find interesting and would love to know the answers to.

Choose the question that vibrates most strongly and sparks off excitement inside you. You will find answers coming and you'll have to scramble to find a pen and paper, or open a Word document quickly. Even though writing something down is supposed to be better for the creative brain, I type fast and love to let it all spill out onto the screen. Choose what works best for you.

Enjoy the awesome results you create with your beautiful mind. This is the real you coming out. Embrace her, welcome her and most of all, listen to her words of wisdom for they will bring you everything you've ever dreamed of.

Day 24
Addressing binge cravings

I have a suspicion that food binges are quite common. I used to cling to that thought when I was considering whether to follow yet another impulse to stuff my face for an hour of sweet oblivion; *Well, loads of other people enjoy these foods, so why shouldn't I? I'm not the only one.*

That may be the case, but did I want to join all those overweight, unhappy people? And I knew it wasn't a smart way to behave. Not only for physical health, but as a beneficial way to deal with feelings and emotions.

So why do we binge? I'd say it is not from physical hunger, not often anyway. For me it was a feeling of escapism, of numbing out and forgetting the world for a little while. A chance to relax and put my own desires first without thinking about anyone else.

In the past, when I had a craving for food that wasn't healthy and wasn't at meal-time, I would mostly give in. It was easier than the uncomfortable, unsatisfied feeling I had as an alternative. I knew this wasn't the answer though. I knew that to stop the cravings, I had to stop giving in to them. By continuing as I was, I was giving cravings the green light to carry on.

It certainly was fun at the time, enjoying all the sweet treats I knew weren't good for me. They were like forbidden fruit, which made them taste even better. But afterwards, it did not feel good. I felt unwell, remorseful and like I would never grow up and be a normal-eating adult. I was like an out-of-control child eating kiddie party treat foods.

What happened when I did not give in

In this chapter, I detail what happened when I *didn't* give into a binge craving, which was the start of a big change for me. If you have cravings too, I hope you find my story useful.

On the day I said *No* to the binge craving, it was hot and humid. I had a day off work and was at home by myself. Normally I would love this, because I can enjoy time to relax, potter, tidy, read and create. I had a slight headache from the weather and my head felt stuffy, hot and swollen.

I'd just had lunch but felt hollow and empty inside and like I could consume tons of junk – sweet food and popcorn, because I felt like it would make my headache better.

I have done this many times before and it does not make me feel better. In fact, I would feel a lot worse after a binge on this type of occasion (surprise, surprise). When I've done this in the past my headache is much worse and I can feel my heart racing from all the sugar.

I am grumpy and short with my husband because not only do I feel irritable from the sugar in my system, but I am unhappy with my own actions so I take it out on him.

This time I asked myself what the deal was, to get to the bottom of the feeling. I find that I have the impending binge feeling described above at home (even without a headache, the headache just compounds it) more than I do at work. I feel discomfort at home more and I find this quite odd as I love home – it is my absolute favourite place to be and I am totally a homebody.

The issue is: I think to myself 'there is *so much* to do', that I feel overwhelmed, and I think this is driving me to eat to have something else to do and enjoy without thinking about everything that *could* and *should* be done at home (and to get away from it temporarily). There is:

Outside:
Weeding
Tidying

Planting
Minor maintenance on our house
Washing windows

Inside:
*Have a shower, do my hair, get dressed, put on
    makeup*
Vacuuming and mopping
Dusting windowsills
Washing windows
Decluttering messy corners
*My wardrobe that seems to fill up and look stuffed
    soon after I've organized and decluttered it
    despite me not going shopping*
Empty the dishwasher
Laundry to wash and hang out
Laundry to bring in and fold
Clean bathrooms and toilets
Rotate seat cushions on the sofas
Declutter the utensil drawer
Change sheets and make our bed
*Dust the cobwebs from the ceiling once I find an 18-
    foot stick*
Trim and water my orchid
Put things away

Plus, there are work jobs I could (should) do because
the business is important, it is our income. Tasks such
as updating the footwear website with new styles,
which I can do from home.

Typing out this list makes me see how I can feel the way I do. It feels insurmountable and I sometimes feel that being at work is less stressful because when I'm there I am not thinking about all that I have to do at home – I can forget about it.

And when I get home after work, well, I've done a full day's work so it is okay for me to relax and not think about anything house-related apart from cooking dinner and watering the plants outside.

Part of being at home on my day off is also the opportunity to have free time to create. To write, sew, potter, play and read in my sewing room which also has all my books in it. But knowing there is that giant list hanging over me makes me not want to do any of those things, because there are other more important tasks and I'd feel guilty if I spent that time playing.

So, often I will do neither the work or the play, and escape by going for a walk down to the supermarket ('I have to get dinner'), also buy a giant bag of whatever and sit on the sofa reading a book or watching television and eating (while also feeling guilty for this). I'm like a kid playing hooky.

Instead of going down that road again, I decided not to eat crap and see what feelings came up. I did this by writing everything down. My first thought was *You can't do everything in one day*. Then I said to myself, *Pick three items off your list*. Yes, I was coaching myself!

My three chosen tasks were:

Have a shower because I hadn't had one yet, and take some headache pills too
Make the bed and do a quick tidy
Go and get dinner from the supermarket

Now that was a bit of a danger spot with the way I was feeling (regards buying snacks to eat). What helped me out was a sentence I had in my slimming notebook:

Just because something is permissible, doesn't mean it is beneficial.

So, I can certainly go and buy a big bag of candy and eat the lot for a quick thrill, but is it beneficial to me? No. Not in the short term (heart racing, more of a headache, guilt) and not in the longer term (makes me fat, and sugar causes all sorts of health issues).

Brian Tracy says that successful people have more of a long-term view than unsuccessful people; the longer your view, the more successful in all areas of life you will be.

The extreme example of this is a junkie looking for their next fix or an alcoholic looking for their next drink. Their view ahead may be only one hour. I could add to the one-hour list someone craving junk food (me).

But a more successful person will be looking much further out than that – days, months, years. As a successfully slim person I would be looking at my slenderness and vibrant health in the future, when I decide that I am not going to give into sugar binges.

By stopping and writing this out rather than stampeding to the junk food dealer (I think supermarkets are like drug dealers sometimes with all the addictive and health-depriving rubbish they sell), it has helped me remember the person I want to be. One who lives life in an elegant way, rather than one who is led around by whims and cravings.

I sometimes think, *What if I had a camera on me at all times, would I be eating this?* My husband is very good with not passing comment on whatever I might be eating or drinking; in fact, we both treat each other as grown-ups capable of making our own decisions.

But sometimes, in good humour when I am chowing down on something low-quality he'll say, *Put that on your chic blog* and we both laugh; but deep down I do feel like a fraud, even if I know that no-one is perfect one-hundred percent of the time.

The peace that comes with a congruent character

I want to be consistent with my personal style and the way I live my life; not one person in public and another behind closed doors. It's a worthy goal to aim for and it certainly feels a lot better than the alternative.

So what did I do then? I did the three tasks on my list that I planned to. I walked down to the supermarket (it's not far from our house) and bought only the five items on my shopping list.

I didn't want to browse the yukky stuff aisles. I felt calm, stable and peaceful. This made me so happy to know there is a better option than eating everything, or white-knuckling it and then still eating everything.

This is the first time I can remember having worked my way through a feeling or emotion and actually navigated it with some success. Afterwards, I felt like I could accomplish anything.

Writing my thoughts down helped so much, even though it certainly wasn't easy at the time. It was like I was ignoring someone hammering on the door while I typed. But, I did it. I talked myself over the empty feeling that was going to have me running to the snack food aisle at the supermarket.

The good news is I proved to myself it can be done; and each time will get easier until it isn't a problem anymore. It all comes down to processing what's going on inside my head; those tangled thoughts that want their voice to be heard. Before I learned this, I was ignoring them, covering them up with food which was only ever going to be a short-term solution.

Your *Thirty Slim Days* action tips:

I hope this chapter has given you hope that you can **conquer your cravings**. You don't have to worry about all the future times that you might be tempted; just focus on doing it today. Even doing this successfully once will give you the confidence that it is possible for you too.

Next time you feel a craving coming on that you don't want to give into, because it goes against your goals and **does not align with the woman you desire to be**; re-read this chapter and go through the process. I can guarantee it will be far less fun than eating what you want to eat, but the feeling from the other side is incredible – well worth the discomfort.

Sit and listen to your feelings and thoughts, then ask yourself 'What am I really feeling? Is it boredom, fear, pain, frustration, anger – what?' Talk yourself through it and ask yourself the next question, and the next; as if you were counselling yourself.

Allow yourself to sit with the discomfort and be uncomfortable (it's not physical discomfort although it may feel like hunger). This was one of the hardest parts for me – the discomfort. I wanted to do something to alleviate it – eat!

It is a discomfort of the *mind*, which is almost harder because you can't think 'I'm cold, I'll put a sweater on' or 'I can feel my skin burning in the sun, I'll cover up'. With your mind **you can't see it, but it's worth persevering with** and working it out. For me, it felt like if I didn't, I *never* would; and I didn't want to go through entire life having these crazy binge cravings.

The weird thing is, at the time you think you literally won't survive if you don't satisfy those cravings, but... you will. You will wake up the next day and feel *so proud* of yourself that you overcame that one time, knowing that **you can do it again and again** and one day it won't be an issue anymore.

You victored. You did it.

Day 25
Practical changes to help you be slimmer

Mindset is a huge part of how much you weigh, and that is why most of this book is dedicated to it. But the more practical aspects matter as well – what you are going to eat, your environment and your habits. You will set yourself up for success when you create good routines at the same time as working on your slim mindset.

For me, it's incredible how fast I have made changes when I get my mindset right alongside taking action. It's like something clicked inside me and now I am rocking all those good habits without effort; habits that I used to find so hard to make stick in the past.

What you're going to eat

This is the big question; what it's all down too, isn't it? There are many structured food plans, and some unstructured ones as well. Any of us could be successful on any of them if we had the right mindset; but I also know that we are all different, so some food plans might suit us better than others.

If you choose to go the structured food plan way, there are a lot of different ones around. Many of us that have had a checkered history with diets will run a mile if we see a grid formation telling us what to eat for breakfast, lunch and dinner though. It immediately feels like constriction and bossiness and we rebel against that.

I am in that camp... a little bit. I think if you come across a food plan that makes sense for *you*, it can give you a good reset. It also has to suit your own palette and any specific health needs you might have; for example, I am celiac, so a food plan that relies on filled rolls and sandwiches for lunch is not for me. You may find dairy doesn't make you feel well. You might not like fish. So look at what they recommend before you choose to follow a certain regime.

Weight Watchers is a huge company that has been around for a long time, and I found it taught me about good portion sizes. I also like that most vegetables are eaten freely on this plan.

Another one I like is Bright Line Eating. I took their inexpensive fourteen-day challenge, which is specifically geared towards those who find themselves addictable to certain foods. I found this plan easy to follow and received great results. It also helped calm down my mind and I felt peaceful around food and eating, which is what I have always wanted; perhaps even more than the weight loss.

I also love Anne Barone's *Chic & Slim* books. They appeal to the Francophile and feminine being in me. She makes weight loss stylish, by choosing to adopt habits she picked up while in the company of chic French ladies.

Reading Anne's books introduced the idea that you could change your eating habits for the better by inspiring yourself rather than restricting yourself. For example, a diet plan might tell you to drink black coffee rather than a sweet, creamy coffee because there are no calories in black coffee.

Going by Anne's method I would choose to drink black coffee because it reeks of Parisian Chic (in my mind anyway, I don't bother myself with the facts when it comes to inspiration). I could imagine myself as a lady at a café sipping her black coffee thoughtfully as she writes in her journal. Doesn't that feel more elegant and alluring than a bossy diet plan?

I would definitely recommend Anne's books as supplemental reading if you are a romantic dreamer as I am.

Most of the time though, I go it alone. I like to look to others to get ideas on portions and to reset my meals, and I continue on with my own common sense. I do love to see what other slender, elegant ladies do, so I often observe what and how they eat if we are dining together. I will also sometimes ask in conversation 'what's for dinner at your house tonight?', which is a reasonable enough question here. I love to get ideas and be inspired by my friends.

Along those same lines, if you are interested in what I had to eat yesterday, allow me to share:

First thing in the morning I had a green tea with my writing time.

For breakfast, I had a bowl of fresh chopped seasonal fruit (it's summer here, so I had apricot, plum and peach), with Greek yoghurt and a sprinkle of whole oats. To complete my breakfast I had a homemade soy milk café latte (made with half milk, half hot water).

At lunchtime, I had a big salad with half a chopped avocado and two medium-boiled eggs quartered on top. A squeeze of lemon juice was my dressing, which mixes in nicely with the avocado. I also had some watermelon afterwards.

For dinner, we had roast lamb with roasted pumpkin, carrot and onion. I made mint gravy from the pan drippings and we had steamed green beans and broccoli with it, which I dressed in a dash of olive oil.

After dinner, I had a fruit herbal tea.

And that's it! Three good meals and no snacks. It's taken me a long time to get to this, but now that I'm living it, I know it's not hard. But that's okay, it takes us all our own time to get into good habits.

If you choose to devise your own eating regime, like I did in my *Day 10. Le Regime Chic* chapter; it's a matter of using your common sense to draw up healthy and filling meals for yourself with restricted quantities of the foods that are richer, and even choosing to eliminate foods you know you cannot eat without overeating them. For me these were always junky processed snack foods, so it was no loss to nutrition.

When it comes down to it, most of us know what is healthy and what is not. We know that eating more fresh fruits and vegetables and less or no processed food is good for us. We know that a tiny dab of butter is preferable to huge chunks, or using plastic margarine instead.

Seeing it written down is what makes all the difference. If you plan your own menu in advance and stick to it *no matter what*, you are a success already. It's much harder to make healthy decisions when you are already hungry and nothing is prepared or decided upon.

Your environment

Setting your environment up for success is all about looking for the 'gaps' – those places where you know you fall down. Then, clean them up one at a time.

For me, I commit to not buying any food that I cannot see my slender, elegant and healthy self eating. If I must buy food for other family members, I hide it away so I can't see it (out of sight, out of mind does work) or buy flavours I don't like but they do.

I used to buy chicken-flavoured potato chips for someone else and was never tempted, even though potato chips were one of my favourite snack foods (only the plain flavour though).

If you are buying treat foods for your children, consider whether you are setting them up into bad habits for the future. That's how I came to have an unhealthy relationship with food and eating – I looked upon unhealthy foods as treats because of my childhood. Consider cutting back on snack food purchases and putting in more healthy options that are also treat-like (such as bliss balls rather than candy).

At high school, I remember my best friend's mum did the groceries once a week and only bought one packet of chocolate biscuits (cookies) each time. They were a family of four – mum and dad, my friend and her brother. Once the biscuits were gone they were gone until the next week.

My friend's mum also made muesli bars which they could have as well though. She called them birdseed bars and they were delicious. They had a few chocolate biscuits each, but also a healthier option once the biscuits were gone. I thought this was a great idea.

It doesn't have to be all or nothing – you can upgrade yours and your family's health in tiny increments. Instead of announcing to your children, *We're no longer having chocolate biscuits*, you can simply buy one packet instead of three, and add in some healthier options to have alongside.

By the same token, my friend's mum loved potato chips but also wanted to keep her slim figure (and she was slim), so she would enjoy them once a week on a Saturday.

My sister, who has been tiny her whole life, is doing a marvellous job training her daughters into good eating habits. They are aged ten and eight, and both dislike fast food franchises, believing the tables, chairs and playgrounds to be dirty and the food yucky. Isn't that excellent brainwashing?

They have broad taste palettes because they've had lots of different foods served to them from a young age. My elder niece loved blue cheese when she was a toddler and it amazes me to see both sisters take or leave bowls of sweets or chocolate.

I watch as they choose a piece of fresh fruit over a wrapped mini-chocolate bar. When I was younger I would devour anything chocolate in my path. My sister is passing on her food habits to the next generation and setting them up for a lifetime of good health, with zero food angst and being a healthy weight effortlessly.

I am not quite sure how my sister picked up selective eating habits, whereas I was a food plough considering we both grew up in the same household. Perhaps there is some truth to us all being individuals alongside our early influences.

Your habits

Look at the times when you habitually snack, and think of ways you can fill that time and space with a different habit. For me, it's before dinner relaxing on the sofa, or after dinner. Before dinner I am hungry. I can easily wait until dinner – I am not in danger of fainting – but I tend to snack.

I made two changes which were helpful. One was to bring dinnertime slightly forward, so that we eat about 6.30pm instead of between 7pm and 7.30pm. I also have a tea or coffee plus a bliss ball or piece of dark chocolate soon after dinner. This finishes off my meal so that I don't find myself wondering if I should pop out for ice-cream.

In addition, I have a knitting or needlepoint project by the sofa that I can pull out and do a bit on each night. Having a project means I don't want salty or sticky fingers to dirty my work, so I knit instead of snack while I watch television.

Massaging moisturizer into my feet and hands does the same job – you don't want to eat with your hands if they are newly moisturized.

Also, brush your teeth. If you want to stop eating after your dinner and find it hard to stop nibbling, brush and floss your teeth. The minty fresh cleanness means you are less likely to want to snack, plus you have already cleaned your teeth when it is time for bed. You can happily have an herbal tea without needing to re-brush.

Thinking about it, you could clean your teeth at other times too. I always brush and floss after breakfast and before bed. But if I find after-work pre-dinner snacking a challenge to avoid (which I can do), why not brush my teeth as soon as I get home from work? That would kill any desire I have for a crunchy salty snack, and by the time dinner is ready the mintiness would have worn off. Genius!

I also find it helpful to gently break habits by changing my routines. If I am in danger of nibbling on the sofa, I'll go and do something else for a little while. It might be pottering and tidying up my makeup area, or moving my reading spot to a chair outside or even sitting up on our bed.

I know I will reinforce a habit by doing it more. I can tell myself 'just try doing something new today', and then it ends up being every day. I also know that a habit can fade away until you don't even remember it being a problem, if you change your routine and have other actions be habitual instead.

Your routines

Make it easy for you to be a slimming success by planning your menu, even if it is only one day or one meal in advance, and preparing your food ahead of time. This means making your lunch salad in the morning or the night before. Have lean protein, a ripe avocado, salad vegetables and fresh fruit ready to go.

For dinner, have everything you possibly can pre-done so that there is the smallest barrier possible to you cooking yourself a healthy meal. When I did not do this in the past I would arrive home after work starving and have to start chopping and prepping. More times than I liked we ended up having unhealthy takeaway meals. We used to call it Fun Mondays when we both arrived home from work at the beginning of the week starving and tired, so would order a pizza. But it was no fun feeling frumpy and fat from low-quality junk food.

I always thought that the vitamins leaked out of vegetables if they were cut too soon, so that was my excuse for chopping right on dinner time. But a few leaked vitamins from preparing my dinner vegetables the night before or in the morning before work was still preferable to a high-salt, high-fat takeaway meal which was my alternative. And really, is leaked vitamins even a thing? It sounds like a big old excuse to me.

Nowadays I am in the habit of automatically thinking ahead to the next meal. I make sure we have everything we need in the fridge and give myself time to prepare it.

Have some form of movement be in your routine also; it doesn't have to be formal exercise. Housework counts, walking to the shop to pick up milk counts, even walking around the supermarket adds steps to your day because many supermarkets have a huge area to cover.

Because I spend so much time writing at my desk, I spread my jobs out throughout the day. I'll write for an hour then make the bed. I'll write a bit more then hang the washing out. I'll sit down for lunch then clean the bathroom. This routine works for my lifestyle and it means I don't sit for hours at a time, and I get all my jobs done too.

Your *Thirty Slim Days* action tips:

Your food

Ask yourself what kind of eating plan (or non-plan) would feel best to you and start following it if it feels good for you to do so. Starting a food plan because you 'know you should' is not a great frame of mind to be in – you will likely self-sabotage yourself from day one.

Instead, get yourself into such an excited state that you can't wait to start eating healthier. This is what I did. I was so enthused by the new healthy me that I cut out unhealthy foods effortlessly. I kept the vision of the new me in mind and she is still leading me. She helps me make good decisions and be enthusiastic about my health and slenderness. She is a star!

Your environment

Consider what parts of your environment, whether at home or work, are detrimental to your goals. Is there someone at work who always brings in yummy treats that you cannot resist? Look the other way (it works!) and tell yourself 'that's not my food'. If you have to be around such food, say *That looks amazing, but I'm so full after lunch. Thanks anyway.*

Is your pantry cluttered and it's hard to find ingredients you know you have? Spend an hour sorting it out and set up your chic and slender pantry instead. Throw out expired food, give away or hide snack foods that you don't want to see and be tempted by. Putting snack foods in a container you can't see through or even stored in another room is a good idea if you have family members who eat foods that are problematic for you.

Your habits

Brainstorm ways that you can disrupt some of your unhelpful habits. A habit is fine if you enjoy it and gain good results from it; however, if a habit is fun but detrimental, find out how you can change your environment, so that you don't have to say *No* to yourself too often – manage those habits out so you won't even notice that they're gone.

It's as if instead of leading a child down the supermarket confectionary aisle and saying *No, you can't have these*, you are walking them past the fresh produce and asking which colour apple they would like. *Distraction*. It can be that easy.

Your routine

Come up with some simple routines that will support you in your journey to living a slim and healthy life. Could you have a chop-a-thon on Sunday afternoon, preparing five lunch salads and all your dinner vegetables for the week? Note down anything that will make life easier for you and reduce the barriers to you choosing healthy foods.

Are there two or three times a week where you can do some form of movement? Stretches before bed, a family park walk on the weekend, swimming in the summer, press-ups against the kitchen counter each morning while the kettle is coming to the boil. You don't have to join a gym to move your body.

Day 26
Create high/low frequency inspiration

I have found that identifying whether an activity or habit has a high or low frequency is a very helpful tool to have on my journey towards becoming and staying slimmer. Nature has given us an inbuilt GPS system which will guide us towards making better choices more of the time *if we only listen to it.*

I read a quote that said motivation is like a lamp which you need to keep putting oil in to keep it going, and I do think this is true. You constantly need to remember your goals and what you want, otherwise the old familiar and cozy habits sneak in again.

But how do you know what constitutes a high or a low frequency? It's so easy that you might dismiss it: You ask if something feels good to you. That's it. Not if something feels good right now, because of course it might feel good to eat a whole bar of Cadbury chocolate at once, but afterwards? Not so good.

For a start there is the physical discomfort. What starts out as a sweet and delicious taste that you want more and more of, becomes a feeling of pain once you have finished the whole bar; crumpled packaging lying nearby.

You also have the remorse at what you've done. You've gorged yourself yet again! *What's wrong with me*, you ask yourself, *that I can't eat like a normal person?* You tell yourself, *I'll never be able to get through life without doing this, I'm stuck with this terrible habit forever and it will be the finish of me! I'll always been fat and I may as well give up and face it.*

Now let's go back to the question 'Does this feel good to me?' *Well it did when I started eating the chocolate,* you think, *but now, no, it does not feel good at all.* The not-good feeling continues on through the week when your scales show a higher number and your clothes feel snug.

Let's rewind time (wouldn't that be a nice thing to be able to do) and bypass the large-size dairy milk chocolate bar at the supermarket. Because even though we tell ourselves that we'll have two squares each night, we know that we are only kidding ourselves. We will actually eat most if not all of the bar in one evening, maybe over two evenings if we start feeling too sick.

So let's go back and instead choose... something different. Maybe we choose a bar of high cacao chocolate that we know we don't eat obsessively. We really are happy with one or two squares with our coffee of an evening.

Or maybe we go into a specialty chocolate shop and choose one exquisite chocolate. We quiet the voice in our head that is telling us 'but you can get the large-size dairy milk bar for the same price as one measly chocolate!'

You ignore that voice and pay for your one chocolate, taking it home in its tiny bag.

Or, you might not buy anything, instead deciding that you're the new slim-girl who doesn't eat sweets much, and prefers to finish her dinner with a black coffee. You feel good thinking that and look forward to starting this new slimming habit.

After dinner, whether you have had your square of dark chocolate, one artisan chocolate or simply a coffee by itself – you feel fantastic. You are happy with your decision; you feel especially happy that you've carried through with it and you feel happy the next morning when you don't wake up with a stomach ache or having put on two pounds overnight.

My after-dinner chocolate habit is one example of creating my own feeling of high (or low) frequency by deciding which choice I am going to go with. Sometimes it really is a split-second decision; so, I catch and remind myself that this choice isn't only for now, it has further reaching consequences as well.

I started putting together a list so I could refer to it, of my own examples of high and low frequency. Then, when a decision came up that needed making, I could remind myself which side it fell on. I didn't end up referring to my lists much at all; the simple act of creating them helped me choose better in the future.

Having high- and low-frequency comparisons is helpful in another way too: simply put, you want *everything* around you to be of a high frequency. It will help you build a successful, stylish, slim and happy life that you adore.

You will see why when you read through my lists below, because each list has their own *feeling*, which is what this whole chapter is all about – feeling good.

Fiona's high frequency list

- Having a daily regime of three nutritious meals, no snacking in between
- Drinking a glass of water often throughout the day
- Having one exquisite piece of chocolate after a meal
- Ordering a small-size coffee in a café
- Looking up salad ideas online and coming up with yummy recipes to make for my lunches
- Deciding that I feel like a break, so making a cup of tea and settling in with my book for a half-hour read
- Having boudoir time after we have eaten and cleaned up; where I can read, apply a face mask and journal

- If I feel like screen-time, set myself a time limit – maybe half an hour – and read uplifting material online: positive and inspiring people I follow on Instagram, Facebook or their blogs
- Habitually looking for the good in others and myself; having positivity; smiling more
- Improving my posture by imagining my head is being pulled up by an invisible thread; breathing fully into my diaphragm
- Having general movement that uses both my big and small muscles – imagine I am walking and moving like a dancer
- Having a clean, organized home; especially focusing on the kitchen and pantry to make it easy to prepare healthy and delicious meals
- Keeping my wardrobe as slimming inspiration by having it edited and making tailored adjustments as necessary; not letting frumpy clothes sneak in
- Having exquisite grooming: smooth, moisturized skin; washing and styling my hair every second or third day; light, sheer makeup even if I am not going anywhere
- Being in bed with lights out by 10pm and getting up at 6am

Fiona's low frequency list

- Eating whenever I feel like it and snacking on junky snack foods

- Not remembering to drink water, having other drinks in preference
- Gorging myself on sweets after a meal
- Having the largest size cappuccino (it's better value) and a muffin at a café
- Not feeling like a salad for lunch and making something yummy and stodgy instead
- Deciding that I feel like a break, so finding something to nibble on and retreating to the sofa
- Spending two hours on the computer after dinner looking at nothing important
- Reading junky newspapers online and feeling the life being sucked out of me
- Being negative; moaning to myself about feeling fat; complaining about uncontrollable topics such as the weather; not thinking about how I might sound before I speak
- Slumping, slouching, shallow breathing; having shoulders rolled forward
- Moving in a heavy way, stomping and walking heavily; sitting down in a flomp
- Letting the pantry become untidy; old food hiding at the back of the fridge
- Doing no other grooming than showering: prickly legs, frizzy hair, shiny t-zone
- Going to bed late – 11pm or later – and not wanting to get up when my alarm goes off, so sleeping in

Reading through these lists, can you feel the energy of each one?

When I go through the first list, it feels positive, happy, go-ahead, moving forward, inspired and creative. With the second list, after reading it I feel stuck, stale, down in the dumps, grumpy and like I'm covered in cobwebs.

This naturally makes me want to do more from the first list and less from the second. I can look at those lists when I feel lazy and slovenly and think to myself, *Which feels better to me? Who do I want to be?* And inspire myself to make a different decision, one with a higher frequency. That's exactly why the second list feels so awful, even just to read it – because the frequency is low.

By staying in a high-frequency, you will naturally attract better circumstances into your life simply by the way you are being. Think about it, when you're living your life on the lower frequency side, good things don't pop up out of the blue do they?

But when you're bouncing along through your day, feeling good for no apparent reason (but we know now it's because you are living more in a high frequency than low), that's when unexpected good things happen.

You run into someone and have a great chat with them; you see a magazine cover advertised that inspires a different course of action or new outfit idea from your own closet. You see how nice the salad display looks at the supermarket and are inspired to pick up a few new items to jazz up your lunchtime salads. Now you are really looking forward to a healthy salad for lunch!

This is the way a high frequency draws good circumstances to you – like a magnet.

Your *Thirty Slim Days* action tips:

Create your high- and low-frequency lists and use them to power you along in a beautiful and seemingly effortless way.

Start by noting down everything that you do currently that makes you feel good both when you are doing it and afterwards too – these are healthy and positive habits. Read through your high frequency list often and use the good energy from that list to inspire you in your actions.

Then, list all your habits that you know aren't adding to your life in a positive way. As you go, add a matching (but opposite) item on the other list. That's how you can build both lists at once and have an example each of high and low frequency for the same habit.

If you read through my two lists, you will see that **each habit has the opposite match**. It doesn't matter which side you start with; ask yourself 'what is the opposite of this habit?'

You will also see on my two lists that not all items are directly related to food and eating. I find it helpful not to limit myself just to those, even if I am actively working on my mindset and habits to become and stay slimmer.

This is because I find *everything* in my life has a flow-on effect to another area. When I lazily tie my hair up wet after a shower and don't take the time to dry and style it nicely, I feel lazy in other ways too.

I think to myself *It's no use putting on any makeup, I'll have a no-makeup day.* My frequency is lowered and the sneaky thought comes in, *Let's not go for a walk this afternoon, let's go and buy something fun and snacky instead...*

On the flip-side, say I start blow-drying my hair immediately after my shower and within twenty minutes it is shiny and smooth. I tie it up into a bouncy ponytail and do a five-minute makeup. Feeling great about myself I get a head-start on chopping the vegetables for my lunchtime salad and healthy dinner.

Everything we do is interlaced into some other part of our life, and it all comes from our feelings. If we do everything we can to feel good on a daily basis, we will continue to make excellent decisions. And really, out of everything we want in life, it all comes down to feeling good. It is human nature to seek out ways to feel good, and we can get that good feeling in a high frequency way (which continues) or a low frequency way (which feels good short-term).

When faced with a temptation or a decision, ask yourself, *Which would feel better not only now, but afterwards as well? Which of my choices has the higher frequency?*

Inspire yourself to **'shop' from your high frequency list** more often and you will see a big difference in your health, happiness and wellbeing. You don't have to be perfect about it either – having more than half of your day being made up of high frequency choices is enough to start with – that's right – only fifty-one percent of choices.

You can do that, right? You know you can, and I know you can too. I have faith in you.

Day 27
Use the 'le half' technique

One of my uncles is often ribbed for his grand proclamation a few years back that he was going to lose a bit of weight and planned to do so by cutting his meals in half. He announced this at dinner-time and showed his commitment by sweeping half the food off his plate – all the green vegetables, leaving potatoes and meat.

I mean, why not cut out your least favourite part of the meal, right? But it's not such a bad thought if you go about it the right way. Imagine eating everything you normally do, just a little less.

I have been practicing this for a while now and it's a painless way to cut back. There is no radical menu plan to go on; no entire food groups to cut out; no expensive diet supplements to purchase.

My favourite breakfast is chopped fresh fruit with two big spoonfuls of yoghurt and a sprinkle of raw mixed nuts. Sometimes I wondered if the yoghurt was good for me though. I know yoghurt is considered a health food, especially the type of yoghurt I prefer – unsweetened Greek-style yoghurt.

However I have sinus headaches from time to time and they can be linked to dairy consumption. I wondered if there could be some benefit for me in excluding dairy from my diet. I eat dairy every day, sometimes quite a few times a day.

Even though I knew cutting out dairy could make me feel better, I also felt quite depressed at the thought of no more yoghurt, no more sour cream, no more trim milk in my Earl Grey tea...

Then I had a revolutionary idea, one that contrasted with my old style of black-and-white thinking – halve the dairy. That way I could get used to having less and maybe wean myself off it if I started feeling better because of that change.

Having only nuts and fruit for breakfast felt like I was missing out, so after my bright idea, I happily dolloped out one big spoonful of yoghurt on my fruit which I then topped with raw nuts. It tasted *just the same*.

After we ran out of yoghurt I didn't buy another container straight away, so there was a gap of about a week. Then I started another container and had the reduced amount again. After that container was finished, I ended up not buying any more and now it has been months since I've had yoghurt on my fruit (but I still have milk in my tea).

I felt like I'd discovered the secret to everything. I didn't feel deprived having half the amount I used to, because I was thinking how awful it would be to have none at all. Having half was like a bonus prize when I was expecting none.

You don't need to go the full half either. You could choose twenty-five percent less for example, as your new strategy.

Continuing through my day – I sometimes enjoy a milky coffee at mid-morning and didn't want to give up both the calcium and fullness to get me through to lunch. So instead of having a big mug (I make it myself), I chose a smaller mug.

Just choose small

If we are out somewhere and order a coffee, I always choose the smallest size available now. It's tempting to get the larger (or largest) size for only a dollar more, but I don't really need it. I have the small size and get my taste of coffee, save a little bit of money and ingest less calories. And I've still had a coffee.

It feels more ladylike and chic as well, to sip from a dainty coffee cup rather than swig on a bucket-sized serving.

This technique could be applied to many other foods that you think you 'should' do without. If you always have two sugars in your coffee, try one-and-a-half, then one. Don't cut down again until you get used to the flavour.

I use the 'le half' technique if I have cheese and crackers as a late afternoon snack. When we have guests, I will make a cheese platter with different types of cheese and a selection of crackers and spreads.

When it's just me however, I make myself a small plate, then I don't carry on nibbling. Usually three or four tiny rice crackers with a small slice of cheese on each is sufficient. I have enjoyed my relaxing time and haven't ruined my appetite for dinner.

A great quote that I often tell myself is '**smaller snacks, smaller slacks**'. It's twee but useful, and highly motivating to me.

Just serve half

At dinnertime, look at what you would typically serve yourself and see if you can adjust it to be less without sacrificing enjoyment or fullness. When I serve up a curry or pasta meal, for example; what I think looks like a small serving is actually too big for me. Without fail.

What I do now is serve myself half of what I think I will eat, and either leave the rest in the pan or dish it into a Tupperware container. When I have done this, I have never gone back for a second helping – not once.

It doesn't matter if foods are healthy either; I realized my lunchtime salads were getting ridiculously big by the time I'd added all the ingredients together.

What helped was to pre-chop some of the ingredients and have them in food storage containers in the fridge. That way I could have a little sprinkle of this, a few slices of that and put the rest back for the next day.

This really is the easiest technique to apply straight away to everyday life. When I had toast for breakfast more often, I would have two, sometimes three slices. It wasn't that I needed three pieces of toast; it tasted nice so I went back for more.

One day I had one piece of toast with peanut butter, then my soy latte. It was enough and I was full through to lunch. That's when I realized I could easily cut calories without feeling deprived.

Even if you go through a fast-food drive-through on a road trip, don't feel like all is lost. Simply choose the smallest burger and combo size and don't upgrade to the large combo, *even if it's only a few cents more.*

You are an elegant lady choosing the elegant portion size. I'm willing to bet that once you have finished your meal, you will be satisfied. You may find the lighter not-stuffed feeling strange, but you will probably not be able to say you are still hungry.

Even if the combo upgrade is free, choose the small size. I have seen bus shelter advertising showing a fast-food slushie drink which is the same price for all sizes.

Apart from the fact that a bright blue drink in a plastic cup is not chic, imagine the look on the server's face if you ordered the small-size. 'But don't you want the jumbo-size? It's the same price' 'No thank you, small is fine', you say.

It's good practice not to be swayed by value, but instead to choose the size you actually want. Sometimes I don't even look at the pricing board, say if I am in Starbucks and don't want the temptation to order a giant-size coffee. I just order 'whatever's the smallest size' and go and wait for my name to be called.

One of my husband's friends, whom he has known since childhood is still in as good a shape as he was as a teenager. It's especially puzzling because he regularly eats fast food for lunch. But what my husband told me is that he notices his friend always chooses the six-inch sub roll rather than the foot-long, or chooses the smallest burger combo if he's out to lunch with him.

I'm not saying this to encourage you to eat junk food; fresh fruit and vegetables and good-quality protein is always better for your health. But if you don't have any other choice of meal venue, just choose the smallest size you can.

Remember this mantra, *Choose a small serving, wear size small*. Keeping this in mind stops me ordering a medium or large serving, because I no longer want to wear medium- or large-size clothes.

Lessen the variety

One last observation of this technique is that it is easier to eat less when you have less variety in a meal. Say you're at a dinner buffet which has ten different dishes to serve yourself from. It is highly likely that you would dish yourself up a larger plate than if there were only three dishes. I use this theory at home when I am preparing meals now.

Making a Thai-style stir-fry showed me that this concept is true – after I'd chopped an onion, a carrot, some broccoli, half a red capsicum (bell pepper), a handful of green beans and added them to the chicken cooking, then served with rice and a tangy Thai sauce, the meal was huge. Despite myself I would continue eating.

Now, I choose two or three vegetables to have with my stir-fried chicken or beef and the quantities are much more manageable. It helps both with serving sizes and how much you eat.

This concept is also well illustrated with a box of chocolates. If you are given a selection box with many different types, you will be tempted to try different flavours and it's hard to stop.

But if you have a box of caramel chocolates, all exactly the same; when you've had one you know all the flavours. I'm not saying it's easy to stop at one, but I think it's easier than if there were many different flavours.

Your *Thirty Slim Days* action tips:

Consider serving yourself less, knowing that you can go back for the rest. Could you do half, or three-quarters? Imagine cutting back by one-quarter with everything you eat or drink. You may barely notice the difference, but over time you would be taking in **twenty-five per cent less calories**.

Make a simple decision that from now on you will be choosing the smallest size for anything you buy or order. Don't calculate the best value, just make it easy on yourself and ask for the smallest size.

It's better this way because **you only need to make the decision once**. You can always go back and buy another small serving – oh, the extravagance! – but I promise you that it is most unlikely you ever will.

Day 28

The magic of slimming affirmations

Anything we can see about ourselves originally started as a thought. Over our lifetime we have built up beliefs about every area of our life. Mostly they are from our immediate family, because these are the people most of us spent the majority of our time with growing up.

We start to absorb others opinions at a young age. If we don't intentionally look at them, we will play them out through our life without even realizing they weren't ours in the first place.

We cannot erase those old, often false, thought patterns; but we can overlay new thoughts over top which, in time, will change how we behave. When I came across this concept and had it confirmed by many different sources all saying the same thing, I felt like I'd had to key to the castle handed to me.

I immediately started examining all the thoughts I had around my constant struggle to avoid unhealthy snack foods which left me in the slightly-frumpy category of body shapes. My beliefs and daily thoughts, which shaped the way I ate at the time, were along the lines of:

It will be no fun to eat only healthy foods
I deserve to have treats each week
It's not realistic to expect me to have nothing sweet after a meal
Others eat a lot worse than I do, why should I change
I don't want to change the way I eat, I like it
I eat mostly healthy meals, I should be allowed snacks

Clinging to these beliefs gave me a tortured existence, even though I knew they were excuses and sounded like a whiny child. Thinking these thoughts about the foods I knew were the root of my problems with weight, health and happiness kept me at a weight that I was never happy with. Yet I didn't want to give up my treats.

Either I had to accept my body shape, health and the way I ate, or I had to change my mind about what I wanted. I couldn't have both. I couldn't eat all of those foods that I enjoyed and have a healthy, slim body too. I couldn't eat as much sugary stuff as I wanted and feel good about myself. I couldn't eat snack foods and look nice in my outfits.

After finding out that I could change my thoughts by reading positive affirmations written in the present tense, I started my own list. I wrote these affirmations to change the way I thought about eating, food and weight.

I would read through this list often, at least twice a day, when I needed it. Sometimes I'd only read part of the list for a quick dip, and sometimes I'd start reading in the middle to give the words a freshness to my mind.

As I read, I would occasionally speak them out loud if I was by myself, and I would feel the emotion behind them. I would imagine that that statement really was true and how good it would feel.

I hope you find these affirmations helpful. Many of them are general so you can read them to yourself while feeling that good emotion. Feel as if each statement was true for you as you read. Having positive emotions in your mind while you read affirmations helps them be accepted by your subconscious in a beautiful way.

You can add affirmations of your own to suit your situation, and you can always start a completely new list if you want customized affirmations to reflect your own issues, challenges and dreams.

You may find as you read that you feel a resistance to certain affirmations. Some may feel too far removed from where you are now. Don't try and talk yourself into believing them, just let them pass by as you continue through the list, and the resistance will fade. Tell yourself that you are not trying to convince yourself of their truth; you are merely enjoying reading them because they sound soothing.

Let's start!

I am choosing to change my size and shape.
I am in control of everything I think.
I am in full control of everything I eat.
I find it easy to be slim and it's now my default.
I love to eat healthy foods and don't like the stodgy stuff anymore.
I am so slim and healthy now and other people have noticed – I can tell they are impressed.
It's been months since I even thought about eating bread; it doesn't interest me anymore.
After streamlining my wardrobe and becoming skinny, I love getting dressed every day now.
I look ten years younger now that I'm skinny.
My clothes drape off me like a model and I love it.
I love fitting all my clothes and that everything looks 1000% better on me.
I am so proud of myself – I have achieved an amazing and permanent result by changing the way I think.
I love going on holiday because I still eat moderately and with pleasure like when I'm at home.
No matter what situation I am in, I am always the same type of selective eater.
I feel physically comfortable with myself today and always.

I feel happy with myself more than I ever have.

I feel strong and capable every day of my life.

I feel good about myself all the time now that I eat normally.

I have clearer thinking now that I am not focused on food or weight loss all the time.

I am looking after my body and it looks after me.

I have healthy cells and an improved immune system.

I forget about food most of the time and am excited to eat healthy when I do feel hungry three times a day.

I feel vibrant and energetic more than a person half my age.

I feel youthful and don't even think about how old I am because it doesn't matter.

I feel younger every year.

I am slowing down the aging process every day.

I sleep well every night and wake refreshed and happy – and skinny.

I used to think it would be a dream come true to wake up skinny – and now I do.

I love the empowering feeling of having internal motivation – it's far more powerful than anything else.

I am so proud that I have realized the vision of how I want to live, be and look.

I love using self-discipline as a loving way of caring for myself.

I feel excitement around being slim and healthy which inspires me every day.

I use enticing reminders of how I want to be, such as motivating photos of celebrities and my favourite inspiring movies.

I love eating simple and clean foods that nourish and support my body.

I drink water regularly throughout the day and can't do without it. My body and my skin feels so good hydrated like this.

I love dressing for winter being slim – I wear skinny pants and boots, a cosy top and big looped scarf. I look amazing!

I enjoy eating a piece of fresh fruit each day and miss it if I don't have it.

I enjoy eating a decent portion of lean protein at each meal.

I enjoy eating salad at lunch and vegetables at dinner.

I miss vegetables when we are on holiday and look for them at any place we eat at.

I feed my body quality foods that it recognises and can utilize fully.

My portions have sorted themselves out effortlessly.

My weight has dropped without effort to the perfect level for me.

I sleep 8-9 hours every night and love going to bed early.

I love wearing all the clothing I own and looking fabulous in every piece.

I love that I am saving money by being slim and healthy.

Processed foods do not interest me anymore.

My fridge, freezer and pantry are a streamlined vision
of yummy and healthy foods.

I am always in control of what and how I eat.

I am in full control and cravings can't touch me.

I am in total control of every thought I think.

I love drinking a big glass of water when I think I am
hungry between meals.

I no longer snack between meals.

I love having three meals a day and nothing else.

I am effortlessly slim today and always.

Why not me? I can be skinny too – proper Paris
skinny.

I love being slim and disciplined, while still being fun
and easy-going.

I choose to drink green tea and I love the taste of it.

I am thin and healthy.

I am in the best shape of my life and it's permanent.

I love the changes I see in myself both in weight and
state of mind.

I love every part of this process and especially my
changing taste palette.

I love doing housework for exercise with my favourite
music playing.

I embrace my health.

I am indifferent to unhealthy foods that I used to love,
and know they are not interesting to me anymore.

I eat healthy and I love it.

My body knows what I like to eat and I listen to my
body.

I choose to weigh 61 kilos and am in love with the way I look and feel.

I always look for the healthy option and if there isn't one, I happily wait until my next opportunity for a healthy option.

I fully trust myself when it comes to food, because I have committed to change.

Days, weeks, months and years go by and I realize I've not eaten or even wanted any unhealthy foods.

I like three meals a day and enjoy feeling hungry before meals.

I don't want extra food between meals anymore.

I find it easy to change.

A sweet tooth is not real, it's an old false story.

I love my big salad for summer lunch, soup and salad in the winter, scrambled eggs too.

I have lots of energy and motivation.

I love my smaller bust.

I love my svelte mid-section.

I love my tiny ribcage and waist area.

I don't eat to bring back memories anymore and it's easy to do.

I remember good times with fondness without becoming overweight.

I find comfort in hot tea, a good book, and a cat cuddle; not food.

The less sugar I have, the less I want; and I don't want any now.

I love that I look and feel 1000% better than I used to.

I never thought I could look so slim and amazing but I do now. I can scarcely believe it, but it's true.
I love to get dressed in my beautiful clothes now, because everything looks amazing on me.
I much prefer looking and feeling amazing, to eating crap.
My clothes drape off me like I am in a fashion magazine spread.
I love that I look much younger than my age now.
I love that my physical age is much less than my actual age.
I care about being slim and healthy because it's good for my health (physical and mental), good for my self-worth and also my self-esteem.
I love the relaxed feeling of being slim.
I love not feeling self-conscious.
I love my fantastic legs, shapely ankles and slender feet.
I love my slim thighs.
I love my small hips.
I love my flat stomach and tiny waist.
I love my modest bust (still bosomy though).
I love curling up on the sofa with a slim torso.
I love feeling dainty.
I love fitting everything I own and looking amazing in it.
I love being a smaller size.
I love people noticing how slim I am.
I love seeing photographs of myself now.

I love the confidence that comes with being slim and healthy – it's good for all areas of my life.

I find it easy to leave old unhelpful habits in the past, because I know now that I have full control over all of my thoughts and therefore my actions.

I am showing my body respect and compassion and it repays me a thousand-fold.

I am a slender success story.

I feel so healthy and skinny and full of vibrant energy.

I love looking good in my chic wardrobe.

I find it so easy to eat only healthy foods.

I love my impeccable posture and find that it's no effort to be straight and tall whether I am sitting or standing.

I love being as slim as I desire and feeling healthy – there is no food that tastes better than this feeling.

I feel vibrant every single day.

I feel empowered refusing foods I know my body doesn't like.

I love being 61kg.

I feel peaceful around food and eating, and more peaceful in general – this is such a change from the past and I am in love with the feeling.

I feel balanced and in control effortlessly.

I eat three healthy meals a day and never think to snack.

Mealtimes sometimes come as a surprise to me and it's only then that I realize how hungry I am.

My stomach always feels comfortable and my torso feels trim – skinny in fact.

I am always aware of how different foods and drinks make me feel, and this helps me decide what to eat.

Life is exciting and fun since I turned my back on rubbish foods. I thought they were my friends but they weren't – they were frenemies!

I love to exercise – I walk every day and I look forward to it.

I enjoy doing my ten-minute weight bearing workouts and stretching exercises on alternate days.

I love eating salad for lunch.

I love eating steamed vegetables and a light home-cooked dinner.

I love drinking lots of water, herbal tea and green tea.

I find it easy to have one drink with dinner and not want another.

I love the taste of a cool and refreshing glass of water and I drink a glass many times every day.

I love a minty fresh, just-brushed mouth.

I love to feel light.

I love weighing 61kg with ease.

I love that every outfit I try on looks great.

I love the fact that healthy and slim people look more youthful.

I love looking skinny.

I love feeling skinny.

I love my curved-in waist.

I love my slim stomach.

I love my slim hips.

I love my nice, slender thighs – they are so trim.

I love that my clothing feels loose.

I love shaving my legs and putting on lotion afterwards because my legs are so shapely.

I love my skinny square shoulders.

I love my defined, angular jaw-line.

I love my awesome cheekbones.

I love feeling hungry before dinner and really enjoy eating my nice home-cooked meal.

I am happy to be alive.

I am happy to be at my dream slim weight now.

I love my life.

Day 29
Twelve mini-techniques

This chapter shares my favourite mini-techniques to help with a fun and enjoyable journey towards slimness and good health.

I hope you find some useful nuggets in them!

An easy life versus a successful life

There is a quote I love which is about an easy life versus a successful life. The old and familiar habits route gives you an easy life because it requires no effort. A successful life feels much better but it requires effort. Most of us want to go the easy route but it is actually harder later on; the route that is harder now will make things easier later on.

For example, it would be easy to eat whatever you want, sit on the sofa snacking every night watching television and never doing any exercise. However, later on you will likely suffer health consequences from obesity and a sedentary way of life, and not enjoy your later years because you have effectively disabled yourself.

The opposite to this – the successful life – means you would go against what other people, advertisers and society tells you is fun. You choose to eat fresh foods, exercise a few times a week and keep yourself healthy. Later on you would reap the rewards of your good habits by enjoying a fit and happy retirement where you travel, socialize and generally love your life.

It's a matter of choosing today which future you would like to live in. Will you choose an easy life or a successful life?

Decide how you want to feel

Think of the saying 'what you resist persists'. By focusing on losing weight, weighing more than you want to and trying not to eat all the foods that have been your comfort in the past, you are focusing on what you don't want.

Focusing on what you *do* want can be hard though, especially when it all seems so far away. It's hard to focus on being slim, feeling on top of the world and how your clothes will look on you when you are skinnier; when you are confronted with the day-to-day realities of your body.

When you feel like this, throw every other thought out the window and focus on how you want to *feel*. For me, I always choose *peaceful*. From the outside I don't seem to look like I have food issues, but the truth is I was always quite angsty and obsessed. My sweet tooth seemed to rule my life and I was often thinking about what I could eat next.

By focusing on the feeling I want in my life which is peace, I feel grounded. I can ask myself 'How can I feel peaceful?' It feels so good to be in this space and I remind myself of it often which brings my focus back to peace. Doing this means I think a lot less about overeating, eating between meals and sugar cravings. It's almost magical.

Next time you are all wound up and feeling like you're never going to get it, think of how you'd rather feel instead. Peaceful? Calm? Soothed? Repeating a word such as *Calm* to myself and letting the feeling wash over me feels wonderful. I can feel my shoulders drop, muscles relax and my forehead soften.

It's almost like you've taken a tonic but it's a tonic of the mind, which is just as powerful.

Detach from the outcome

Whether it's becoming slimmer or anything else you wish to achieve, consider detaching from the outcome. What I mean by this is that if you are so focused on your goal weight, you can become demoralized if you still have some way to go. It's easy to think that healthy eating day-by-day isn't going to do anything.

The key to success in any endeavour is to detach from the outcome and immerse yourself in the process. I know that all sounds a bit business-speak, but when it's applied to becoming your desired weight, it means to stop fussing over the scales every week and instead focus on one day at a time. Focus on what you are going to eat *today*. Focus on the process of becoming slimmer.

For me at one stage it meant stopping my regular weigh-ins and just focusing on my healthy meals, no snacking and no sugar. I continued with my slimming notebook and wrote all my meals down, but I didn't write in my weight because I wasn't weighing myself. When I went back to the scales, I loved the number I saw.

When you find your mind wandering off to worry about something in the future, bring it back to *today*, and what you are going to do *today*. Removing the thought of whether you can achieve your goal weight makes it easier to focus on what you can control right now – what you are feeding yourself.

Make it hard to snack

Resist stocking up on special deals or buying goodies just in case. I made this a rule and it works well for me. Now, if I get a craving, it's a lot more difficult to get my fix. Most of the time I will ride it out, either having nothing, or a glass of water or cup of tea. Sometimes I will eat a snack, but it's much healthier than I might have had with my favourite treats in the house.

There is the odd occasion that I will go out and get something and yes, I do indulge. But those times are far fewer than they used to be.

It's like they say about having good security on your home. If a burglar wants to get in, they'll get in, but if the house looks too secure they'll likely go looking for an easier target. It's the same with your repeat offender snacks. Keeping a supply at home will make snacking on them an easy target.

You will effortlessly cut down your consumption of them if you store them *at the supermarket* or wherever you buy them from, instead of down the hall or in the next room.

In addition, being a thrifty girl, it hurts me to pay full-price for something when it's on special every other week; so this also cuts down on my supermarket snack purchases.

Gather inspiration from others

I always note when something sparks a little germ of excitement inside me. Maybe it's somebody being quoted in a magazine about how they maintain their slim figure, maybe it's how they have lost weight and kept it off, or maybe it's their excellent attitude towards food and eating. If something really speaks to me, I'll save it.

If I'm in a waiting room with a magazine, for example, I will take a photo of that paragraph with my phone. If it's a Facebook or Instagram post I will take a screenshot. If it is an online news article or blog post I will copy and paste. I used to write little bits in a quote book, but now I mostly save these snippets in a Word document called *Fiona's Slimming Inspiration*.

Compiling these little oddments of excitement and inspiration into one Word document means that when I go back to it, it's like my very own custom designed reading material to re-inspire me. I used to print these documents out and put them in clear-files to read at home (you can get binders with clear plastic pages to slip documents into), but now I use my Kindle for this.

I love to make my own eBook inspiration by emailing Word documents to my Kindle (you are given a Kindle email address when you buy one). If it is a document that I update with new material, like my inspiring quotes document, I simply delete the old document from my Kindle and send the new version to myself.

In this document, I include whole or part of an online article or blog post as well as quotes and snippets. Mostly I keep everything and add to it, but every so often I will delete a part that no longer resonates with me.

Why not curate your own inspiration to keep your vibration on an elevated level?

Put some chic into it

Act as if you were your ideal self and ask her what she would eat on a normal day.

How would she feel about herself, and how would she do self-care? Would she take a book and sit in the park reading instead of going to a café and having cake? If she did meet friends in a café would she have a black coffee with no food?

Channel her and make it seem fun and fashionable to yourself instead of 'moan, moan, I can't have cake because I am dieting'.

Which sounds like a more elegant and enticing way to approach slimming to you?

Reframe your actions

When I started weighing and measuring my food and sticking to strict portions in an effort to reset my eating habits (because I knew my portion sizes had become too large), I felt silly. I felt like a stupid person who didn't know how to eat after more than four decades on this planet. This feeling almost made me give up on the first day of my new regime.

Then I thought about fitness professionals and body builders. They weigh and measure their food and stick to strict menu plans all the time, because they are going after good results in their physique. They aren't stupid or pathetic having to be told how to eat. They are simply serving themselves foods and portions that will get them the results they desire.

At the time, reframing my new food regime to 'this is how fitness professionals do it' helped me feel better about weighing my dinner before I ate it. I felt in control and proud that I was doing the same things they were.

Shift your focus

Don't fantasise about the food you are not having on your healthy eating regime. I remember years ago falling to sleep one night imagining how a fairy cake with whipped cream would taste. I didn't even really like them, but because I was eating healthy and hadn't had a 'treat' in eons, I was fantasising about this fairy cake!

This is not great for your mind, because what you focus on grows. You will be drawn back to unhealthy foods and eventually end up eating them and finding yourself back to how you were before.

Say a food thought pops into your mind, maybe it's chocolate-covered Scorched Almonds you see a magazine advertisement for. Seeing this advertisement reminds you how much you love them, *Gosh they'd taste nice...* Stop right there! No good can come from this. You are only talking yourself into caving in, and there is an alternative.

Instead, as soon as you find yourself gazing at the picture of ice-cream or dreaming about chocolate, switch your thoughts to luscious, healthy foods. A shiny red apple, crispy salad, a cool and refreshing mouthful of chilled sparkling mineral water.

Instantly you will find your mind is reset and all unhealthy food thoughts have simply been brushed aside. Dwell on what you want to be in your future.

Surround yourself with luxury

Once or twice a year my husband and I spend a night at our favourite five-star luxury hotel in the city where we live. They often have special offers and package deals and we book one of those.

We go for a swim in the roof-top pool after we've checked in, lounge around our room in big white fluffy robes, dress for drinks at the bar and enjoy gourmet foods at dinner.

The rooms are sumptuous and the experience is well worth the price for us. It costs about the same as a fancy dinner out. We never fail to return home refreshed and re-inspired to upgrade our daily life.

One of our visits gave me the idea to create our daily meals as if we were guests at that hotel. We could enjoy our resort-style breakfast of fresh tropical fruits and coffee, dine on fresh-caught fish in the evening and have all our foods be simple, fresh and top-class.

By doing this not only were we upgrading our choices, but we were investing in our health. 'Put your money where your mouth is' is literally true in this case.

It didn't cost us a fortune either, in fact our grocery bill has stayed the same.

I used to think that some grocery items were too expensive so wouldn't buy them, yet would fill my trolley with cheap snack foods. What a back-to-front way to think!

By looking down on the junky milk chocolate (they'd never serve *that* in a five-star hotel), I could easily replace it with a smaller bar of 90% cacao chocolate that I could enjoy one or two squares of.

There is even a price to pay with cheap junk food – you end up paying for it in other ways – non-monetary ways such as feeling revolting after eating it and feeling bad about yourself; as well as monetary ways such as not being able to fit your clothes so you buy more, and the cost of visiting a doctor because you have health issues caused by unhealthy eating. There are a lot of hidden costs to cheap junky food when you think about it.

The key to becoming slim and healthy is to buy delicious and healthy food that you look forward to. Design your own five-star resort-style breakfast. Find delicious extras such as spiced dukkah mix to sprinkle over your lunchtime salad.

I have a yummy paleo breakfast mix that I buy. It's expensive but I only use one spoonful over my fruit each morning. The bag lasts for weeks. And I was not buying that initially, but spending money on junk. Something was not adding up.

The bonus is, that an upgrade in one area of your life will spill over into other areas of your life, influencing them favourably as well: 'a rising tide lifts all boats'.

How can I?

I love the *How Can I* game. It's a fun way to journal and it all starts with a question that begins with *How Can I?* Decide what you want and then ask yourself that question. Keep writing and see what you can come up with.

Write down all the answers, even silly or unrealistic ones. Here are a couple of mine to get you started off.

How can I inspire myself to... Be 61kg?

Get excited by fashion again
Redo my wardrobe
Feel empowered by my decision to be slim
Absorb my slimming affirmations
Declutter our home a bit at a time – write out a plan and tick areas off
Curate a Pinterest inspiration board – visit it at least once a day and feel excited for when I look the same
Read weight loss success stories such as in Weight Watchers and other slimming magazines (plus on their website) – be inspired by the before and after photos
Read fitness magazines for inspiration

Eat like a body sculptor – protein and good fats, lower
the carbs, lots of water
Keep up my grooming – smooth, shaved, moisturized
legs and underarms
Visualize myself as the health and fitness girl who
effortlessly weighs 61kg.

How can I become and maintain a consistent 61kg weight in a fun, easy and healthy way?

Walk every day
Drink water between meals
Eat water-rich foods such as fresh fruit and vegetables
Enjoy eating in a healthy way
Look forward to meals because I haven't eaten since
my last meal
Sip herbal tea
Get a craft project for when I watch television
Streamline our fridge and pantry
Plan meals
Enjoy a drink by itself before dinner – no nibbles
needed
Feel empowered by being this way
Love the feeling of health and slimness
Try hypnotherapy?
Look forward to going to bed early
Map out three twenty-minute weight-bearing
workouts each week (google hotel room workout
or military workout)

Some of these statements were factual for me when I wrote them, and some were works in progress; but they were all in the direction I desired to go in. Mingling them together helped them sink into my brain, which reinforced what I wanted to believe and how I wanted to be.

Whatever you immerse yourself in is how you will end up behaving, so why not surround yourself with positive statements and exciting new beliefs. By ignoring all the old thoughts and beliefs, they will fade away into the background. At the same time, you can layer over new thoughts and beliefs and gradually turn yourself into this new person that you desire to be.

It takes time and repetition, and that's okay. You've been the way you are for a long time, so it makes sense. Just keep repeating over and over and one day you'll find... you are that person.

Create good habits

Small habits today can seem insignificant and benign, but in ten years' time they won't be. Habits are amplified by time and will create significant effects either good... or bad.

In my book *Thirty Chic Days* I devote a whole chapter to this concept; it's called *'Little and often'* (Day 18). In this chapter I wrote:

'If there exists a universal rule for life, it could well be little and often. Anything worth achieving is

constructed step by step, brick by brick, habit by habit. We are the sum of our daily routines; these can be good practices that build us up or unhelpful, unconscious patterns that sabotage our efforts.

Anything we do regularly quickly becomes a subconscious habit. As we repeat tasks and thoughts, they become ingrained in our brains much like shortcuts across the grass on a walking route. It's easiest to turn to familiar thought routes which is why it's important to avoid training ourselves into bad habits. By the time we realize they are hindering our efforts towards a beautiful life, these fine threads of thought have turned into heavy chains which are holding us back.'

Consider habits that you have that you suspect might be dangerously small and work out a way to either change them or stretch them out. A chocolate bar every afternoon at work is a great example.

Can you either change that chocolate bar to a bliss ball that you make a batch of every few weeks, having one a day (bliss balls are made from dried fruits and nuts, sometimes with cocoa powder). Or, can you look forward to a chocolate bar on a Friday afternoon instead of five times a week?

With my pre-dinner Diet Coke which I knew was not good for me, I changed it to a glass of Lemon Perrier. I didn't even miss the cola flavour; it was the fizziness that I enjoyed.

Dig out those little habits and try a few ways to address them with the least amount of disruption to your happiness. You will be so happy you did in ten, twenty or thirty years' time!

A quick slim girl swap

I was out shopping for a new summer dress recently, when I realized I was quite thirsty and hadn't had a glass of water for a while. I decided to pop into the supermarket in the shopping centre and buy a big bottle of water. There was a display of 1.5 litre bottles of spring water right inside the main entrance and they were 89 cents a bottle.

I bought one and took a drink. Walking around holding my big bottle of water I felt like a slim Hollywood star; you know how they are *always* carrying a bottle of water in paparazzi photos. I had the thought that this could be a great substitute for a chocolate bar or sweet creamy coffee drink. Of course, if you are craving those things, a bottle of water will not seem appealing, but if you tell yourself you can have something sweet after if you still want it, you likely won't.

You will have quenched your thirst, feel amazing from having hydrated your body and you will probably be surprised that you will have drunk most of the water by the time you get home.

You've still bought yourself something so it satisfies that part of your brain. Nothing kills a craving like having lots of yummy cool, crystal clear water and you haven't taken in any calories. Win/win!

Day 30
You can do it

Now we are nearing the end of the book, I want to remind you that *you can do it*, you really can. You can decide that this time you will commit to doing whatever it takes and keep on going, no matter what.

Reading a book like this and looking at all your habits and beliefs can feel uncomfortable. For me it sometimes felt safer to be in ignorance. I'd tell myself 'Sure, I might not be completely happy with my weight and my eating habits but I'm not *that* bad'.

Before looking at how and why you eat, you were happily in the dark about the underlying messages floating around. Exposing all your habits fully is like discovering a giant mess in the attic. It's tempting to slam the trapdoor shut, but it's still there.

When you start looking into your beliefs and tangled feelings you think 'How am I going to work through all this? I'd almost rather live in ignorant bliss'. It's scary and the rabbit-hole seems really deep.

Just do it gently and incrementally, one little bit at a time with lots of self-love and self forgiveness.

Let yourself be a new person

Even if something upsetting happens, you don't need to fall prey to food. Even if you feel bored and know that something tasty will perk you up. Even if you think 'what's the point, I may as well enjoy myself now'. These are false messages from a little voice inside you that has been sent to test you.

It is common to self-sabotage when the going gets too good. It's almost like we have an upper level on how happy, slim and successful we are allowed to be before we pull ourselves down again. You aren't that way anymore; you know the old saboteur's tricks and you are not falling for them any longer.

I know you can do it, and you do have it inside you; you have the metal to achieve your goals. Don't be tempted by a short-term fix that will set you back and demoralize you.

Don't worry about never eating 'X' again, and how you will cope. You don't have to worry about that; just do what you do *today*. Choose to eat in a healthy and normal way *today*. Make it into a challenge by crossing days off a calendar each day you nourish yourself and make great choices.

Think about your new normal of eating three healthy meals, hydrating yourself with water, and getting good sleep by setting times you will go to bed and get up. The more you practice your good habits, the more normal they will seem.

Changing habits for the better feels strange at first but then you become used to them. Remember what Marisa Peer says 'Make the familiar unfamiliar, and the unfamiliar familiar'. Make it unfamiliar to gorge on foods that make you feel sick.

Reframe how you want to feel on special occasions

Train yourself to move away from the habit of looking at special occasions such as birthdays, holidays and vacations as a reason to let all your healthy ways fly out the window because you want to 'treat' yourself.

It's far more of a treat for your body to enjoy the same healthy foods you have been having all along. Maybe more luxurious versions of these foods would be nice, but don't go back to the same old gut-rot (my dad's word!) that made you so unhappy for all of those years.

My husband and I travelled to Sydney for four nights last year, and I vividly remember one afternoon we stopped at a city supermarket to buy some fruit and yoghurt for our breakfast. When we left, there was a barrow in the mall that had every type of candy known to man. It was a colourful and enticing sight and 'because I was on holiday' I found a bag and a scoop and started pick'n'mixing.

Back at our hotel I happily nibbled away while we spent a few hours resting before we headed out for dinner. I overdid it and can still remember how ill I felt and how uninterested I was in our evening meal. My stomach was full of sweets and I barely touched my dinner. What a waste of a lovely evening.

At that time I thought it was no fun at all to enjoy my afternoon downtime with a flute of sparkling mineral water – *So boring!* but I bet I would have been happier later on, not having filled myself up with terrible things. *C'est la vie*, I live and learn.

I have learned now not to put short-term gratification ahead of feeling well; being in a slim and healthy body and having high self-esteem. It's almost like I gave myself away too cheap for a bag of coloured sugar.

Put your success plan into action

It's fine to be scared and apprehensive about the future, but don't let that stop you from even trying. Your future is made up of *todays*. All you ever have is *today*. All you ever need to do is make yourself proud today and the rest will take care of itself.

Put safety measures into place to ensure you will be okay. Don't buy foods just in case. Make sure your kitchen is well stocked with all the healthy options you need for the week.

Prepare meals ahead of time as much as you can to ensure you don't arrive hungry at your dining table and you still have to chop and cook. Measure portions out, chop your vegetables earlier in the day or the night before. Pre-cook food if that helps. I like to make extra servings of easily reheatable dinners such as meatloaf and savoury mince.

These habits add up, making life easier for yourself which also means you will take the healthy option, because it has now become a default. When you are driving home from work and can smell the pizza place as you drive past, close your mind to it. It holds no interest to you anymore because you are a different person. One who values herself. You also know that you have a wonderful meal ready to go as soon as you walk in the door which will taste far superior to that cheap pizza.

Move your dinner-time earlier if you have to. That's how I addressed my late afternoon snacking habit, by moving our dinner hour from 7.30pm to 6.30pm. Some days if I was feeling famished I'd eat at *6pm*. I know it's not very rock-and-roll or Euro-chic (how do the Spanish manage not to eat until 10pm?) but it was great for my healthy habits.

The unexpected bonus of an early dinner-time was that I now had this lovely long evening to enjoy and still get to bed nice and early. Plus, I wasn't going to sleep on a full stomach which was much more comfortable too. It feels quite pleasant going to bed thinking, *Hmm, I could eat*, because it's been a few hours since your evening meal. Maybe if you get hungry later on, move your evening meal as far *back* as possible.

If after dinner is your problem snacking time, do whatever it takes. Brush and floss your teeth straight after dinner. Read a book rather than watch a program if you have linked television and snacks together. I associated our sofa and a book with snacking, so if I am feeling tempted, I read in the bedroom instead. Apply a face mask and listen to relaxing music. Write in your journal. Knit or crochet. Go to bed early if you're finding it really hard going.

One weekend I found myself craving something sweet and junky after lunch. The cravings were so strong I was afraid I was going to give in to them, but I didn't want to because I knew I'd be back at square one then.

I also didn't have much energy to do anything to distract myself so I lay down on the sofa and had a nap for a couple of hours. I didn't plan it but it ended up being the best thing I could have done in that situation. I had avoided snacking at the same time as giving my body a rest.

Go easy on yourself – you're doing an amazing job

Changing the way you eat and losing weight takes its toll on your body. It's an endurance for sure. You may feel tired some days and you may have a headache as you remove or reduce certain foods such as sugar or caffeine from your diet.

After I stopped sugar altogether I had a dreadful four-day headache. It was horrible. I also felt tired, *so tired*, right from my bones out through to my skin. It was like an aura of heaviness around me.

I'm not sure if it was all from sugar or brought on by the humid weather too, but I hung in there and did not self-medicate with sweets (yes, I used to do that all the time and no, it did not *ever* work).

On day five I felt like a new person. My head was clear, I had good energy and felt so happy to be alive. I felt like I had been reborn. I'm so glad I stuck with it and stepped through that fire-pit to emerge like a phoenix out the other side.

Take notice of your low times of energy and baby yourself. I now know that late afternoon can be a time like that for me. Probably it's why I used to snack then – to boost my energy levels. Now, I try to have all my work down by mid-afternoon, including preparation for dinner.

I then give myself full permission to rest for a couple of hours before dinner. Sometimes it's easy and sometimes I feel like the laziest person on earth. But I get up at 6am and start my work then. I work from home so I feel grateful that I can do that.

When I used to work in a nine-to-five job I would handle this by organizing dinner the night before – not always, but it really helped if I did – or even better still, on the weekend. Not every part of a meal, but even planning what to serve and having the fridge full of provisions was a big help.

If I didn't have dinner planned to be eaten not long after I walked in the door, it was a little bit dangerous. Especially if there was chocolate around.

Do everything you can to gain feel-good momentum

The hardest time is when you first start. You feel like you are depriving yourself and for what? You are still heavier than you'd like to be and you can't eat any of your favourite foods. That sucks!

But if you give it some time and keep your frequency high with all the suggestions in this book, soon enough you will start seeing changes from your new, healthy regime. You will see a difference on the scales. You will start to feel more energetic.

The ball has started rolling and you are gaining momentum. All you have to do is keep on going, and it's easier now because of this. Remember, winners never quit and quitters never win. You are not a quitter, you are a winner.

You will do whatever it takes for however long, because what's the alternative? You don't want to go back to the way you were before; it was awful then. Remember the unhappiness, the unhealthiness, the low feeling?

That crap that big companies peddled to us as fun; it's not worth it, and we both know that. They sucked us in once, but never again. We are wise to their tricks. We know now that nourishing ourselves on fresh, whole foods is the answer to everything. We feel happy, slim and full of vim and vigour. We are unstoppable!

I wish you all the health and happiness in the world. I have faith in you – I know you can do it. Look upon healthy eating as a fun and exciting way to gain everything you ever wanted. Once you upgrade this area, the goodness will spill over into every part of your life. It can't not.

Start today if you haven't already. Start every day. Keep on going – you're worth it! No-one else is going to care as much about you than *you*. You are the one solely responsible for what you eat, even if someone else does the grocery shopping.

You can choose to be different to how you were. You can choose to be different to the people around you. Be the one who shines a light and leads the way; not with your words, but with how you are. Inspire others as well as yourself with your actions.

You can do it. I have faith in you.

Now go out there and be fabulous.

To finish

It is my wish that you have found tons of ideas in this book to put into practice, and I also sincerely hope you have found encouragement. I know how easy it can be to feel discouraged about your weight.

I also know that feeling excited and hopeful about the future is the best way to change things for the better. When I felt like I 'should' do things to be healthier, that's when I dug my heels in. I was rebelling against myself! I mean, why shouldn't I have fun and be skinny; who said it had to be a torture contest?

I have proven to myself that it can be (fun, not a torture contest); it just takes looking at things from different points of view. I hope you can see those other angles now too.

I hope all the ideas, tips and techniques were enjoyable for you to read, and I highly encourage you to go back and do some of the exercises for yourself (not only 'exercise' exercise, but written and thinking exercises as well!) Choose the one that feels best for you to start with.

It's fine to read about interesting ideas, but it isn't until you put your knowledge and own thoughts into action that change happens. Whenever I have done something instead of just reading about it, I have had big breakthroughs and shifts in my thinking that allowed me to make lasting change. *That*, my friends, is exciting to have happen to you.

Above all though, have fun. Don't do anything that makes you feel heavy of spirit. If you do choose an exercise from one of the action tips at the end of the chapters, or decide to do your own version of your perfect day (*Day 2. Start with a vision*), do it because you can't wait to, and feel so excited for the results.

That is my over-arching belief that runs my life for the most part – make what you want to do enticing and fun, then it will seem effortless.

I'd love to hear how you get on, and am always available at:

fiona@howtobechic.com

I look forward to your email letting me know that you are making great strides into your gorgeously slim and healthy life.

All my best to you,
Fiona

About the author

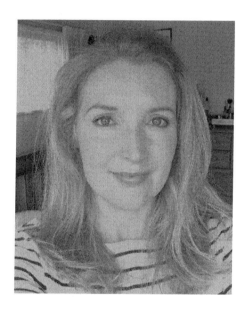

Fiona Ferris is passionate about, and has studied the topic of living well for more than twenty years, in particular that a simple and beautiful life can be achieved without spending a lot of money.

Fiona finds inspiration from all over the place including Paris and France, the countryside, big cities, fancy hotels, music, beautiful scents, magazines, books, all those fabulous blogs and Instagram accounts out there, people, pets, nature, other countries and cultures; pretty much everywhere really.

Fiona lives in beautiful Auckland, New Zealand, with her husband, Paul, and their two rescue cats Jessica and Nina.

To learn more about Fiona, you can connect with her at:

howtobechic.com
fionaferris.com
facebook.com/fionaferrisauthor
twitter.com/fiona_ferris
instagram.com/fionaferrisnz
youtube.com/fionaferris

Fiona's other books

All available from:
amazon.com/author/fionaferris

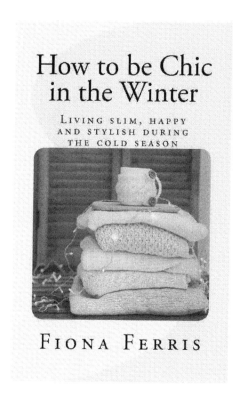

How to be Chic in the Winter: Living slim, happy and stylish during the cold season

Paperback and Kindle

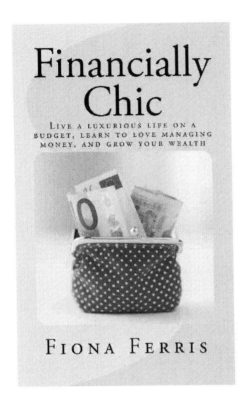

Financially Chic: Live a luxurious life on a budget, learn to love managing money, and grow your wealth

Paperback and Kindle

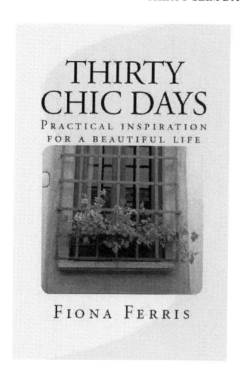

Thirty Chic Days: Practical inspiration for a beautiful life

Paperback and Kindle

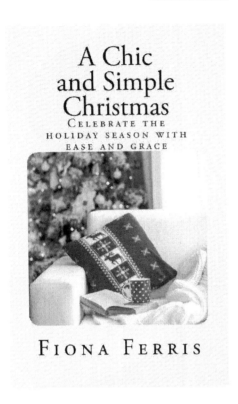

A Chic and Simple Christmas: Celebrate the holiday season with ease and grace

Paperback and Kindle

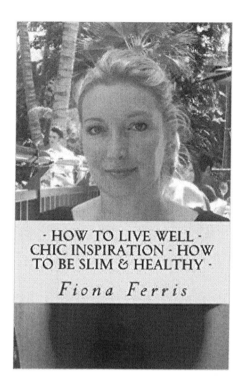

{3 in 1} How to Live Well - Chic Inspiration - How to be Slim and Healthy

Paperback and Kindle

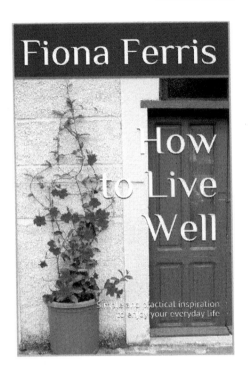

How to Live Well: Simple and practical inspiration to enjoy your everyday life

Kindle only

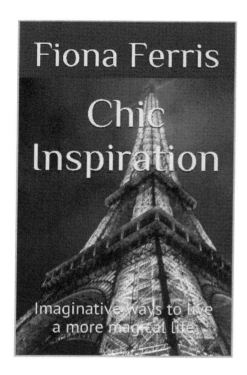

Chic Inspiration: Imaginative ways to live a more magical life

Kindle only

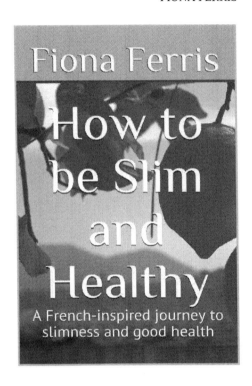

How to be Slim and Healthy: A French-inspired journey to slimness and good health

Kindle only

354

23844245R00208

Printed in Great Britain
by Amazon